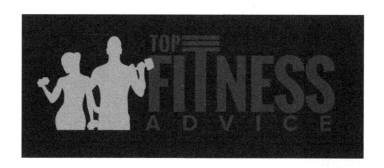

KETOSIS

A Beginners Guide On How The Keto Diet Helps You Lose Weight & Biologically Turn Your Body Into A Fat Burning Machine

LINDA WESTWOOD

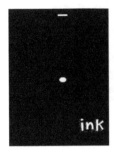

First published in 2017 by Venture Ink Publishing

Copyright © Top Fitness Advice 2019

All rights reserved.

No part of this book may be reproduced in any form without permission in writing from the author. No part of this publication may be reproduced or transmitted in any form or by any means, mechanic, electronic, photocopying, recording, by any storage or retrieval system, or transmitted by email without the permission in writing from the author and publisher.

Requests to the publisher for permission should be addressed to publishing@ventureink.co

For more information about the contents of this book or questions to the author, please contact Linda Westwood at linda@topfitnessadvice.com

Disclaimer

This book provides wellness management information in an informative and educational manner only, with information that is general in nature and that is not specific to you, the reader. The contents of this book are intended to assist you and other readers in your personal wellness efforts. Consult your physician regarding the applicability of any information provided in this book to you.

Nothing in this book should be construed as personal advice or diagnosis, and must not be used in this manner. The information provided about conditions is general in nature. This information does not cover all possible uses, actions, precautions, side-effects, or interactions of medicines, or medical procedures. The information in this book should not be considered as complete and does not cover all diseases, ailments, physical conditions, or their treatment.

You should consult with your physician before beginning any exercise, weight loss, or health care program. This book should not be used in place of a call or visit to a competent health-care professional. You should consult a health care professional before adopting any of the suggestions in this book or before drawing inferences from it.

Any decision regarding treatment and medication for your condition should be made with the advice and consultation of a qualified health care professional. If you have, or suspect you have, a health-care problem, then you should immediately contact a qualified health care professional for treatment.

No Warranties: The author and publisher don't guarantee or warrant the quality, accuracy, completeness, timeliness, appropriateness or suitability of the information in this book, or of any product or services referenced in this book.

The information in this book is provided on an "as is" basis and the author and publisher make no representations or warranties of any kind with respect to this information. This book may contain inaccuracies, typographical errors, or other errors.

Liability Disclaimer: The publisher, author, and other parties involved in the creation, production, provision of information, or delivery of this book specifically disclaim any responsibility, and shall not be held liable for any damages, claims, injuries, losses, liabilities, costs, or obligations including any direct, indirect, special, incidental, or consequences damages (collectively known as "Damages") whatsoever and howsoever caused, arising out of, or in connection with the use or misuse of the site and the information contained within it, whether such Damages arise in contract, tort, negligence, equity, statute law, or by way of other legal theory.

Table of Contents

Disclaimer	3
Who Is This Book For?	7
Introduction	9
What is Ketosis?	11
Ketosis Mistakes and Misconceptions	19
Optimal Foods, Safe Foods and Bad Foods for Ketosis	23
Ketosis' Overwhelming Success	27
What is a Ketogenic Diet?	29
Breakfast Recipes	35
Lunch Recipes	71
Dinner Recipes	105
Conclusion	161
Final Words	165

Would you prefer to listen to my book, rather than read it?

Download the audiobook version for free!

If you go to the special link below and sign up to Audible as a new customer, you can get the audiobook version of my book completely free.

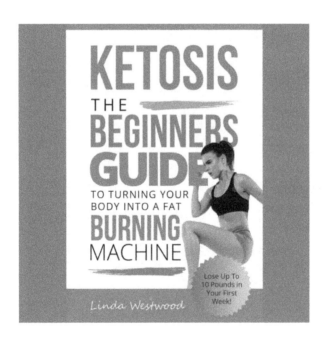

Go here to get your audiobook version for free:

TopFitnessAdvice.com/go/ketosis

Who Is This Book For?

People these days are highly health conscious and therefore can be mostly seen dieting, exercising in the gym or following a strict and specific diet chart for maintaining the health and keeping themselves fit.

But some people in order to keep their body fit tend to skip their meals creating the lack of essential nutrients in their body which many have various adverse effects on them in the future. Such an act reduces the immunity in the body and gives an invitation to numerous diseases making the body weak.

Therefore, people should have a healthy diet plan which not only keeps them fit but also provides the essential nutrients and the maintaining the daily calorie in the body.

Introduction

A healthy diet plan also lowers the risk of heart attack and various other diseases. The healthy diet plan should include fruits, vegetables, milk and milk products, beans, poultry, lean meats, fish, whole grains, eggs and nuts. It controls the meal portion size according to different human beings as every person has a distinct appetite.

If you are aiming to lose weight then the biggest problem that arises is the confusion of what to eat. The diet of a person is perfect if it includes 2500 calories a day like a breastfeeding mother.

A healthy consumption of diets not only helps in reducing the cholesterol, blood pressure, blood glucose but also minimizes the body risk for cardiovascular diseases. It also helps in slowing the progression of any of the diseases if you are following a healthy diet plan containing all the essential nutrients.

So, your diet cannot be completely blamed for your gaining weight, as there are many people who even after eating more remains thin which occurs because of their hormones or genetic factors.

Thanks again for purchasing this book, I hope you enjoy it!

What is Ketosis?

Fat, as a dietary component, continues to be the subject of much misinformation and controversy. Many diets, and even diet fads, have emerged in the past thirty years extolling the value, not only of making fat a regular part of the diet, but making it the major component of our daily nutrition.

Still, detractors of high-fat diets have called them unsafe and even dangerous, as proponents vowed that going on a high-fat diet is the surest way to fast and safe weight loss, and better overall health.

The Ketogenic Diet has been at the forefront of this diet "revolution," and its popularity continues to increase as new scientific evidence continues to surface and prove that fat does not deserve the bad nutritional rep it has received.

Is fat really bad?

Contrary to popular belief, dietary fat is not bad, but there's a reason behind the misconceptions regarding fat – they are brought by years of misinformation partly sponsored by the US Department of Agriculture.

In the "Dietary Guidelines for America, 2015-2020," issued by the U.S. Department of Agriculture, fats are included in the part where oils are mentioned, stressing that food oils are limited to fat in liquid form at regular room temperatures. The guidelines specifically named vegetable cooking oils, and made it seem like oils were the only source of fat nutrients available for human consumption.

Dismissing these "oils" as secretions from fish and plants, the guidelines further pointed out that they do not constitute a separate food group, but exist simply to supply some essential macro nutrients, and on a very limited level, at that.

A "My Plate" diagram from the same USDA report, once again dismisses fat, and shows the "acceptable" five food groups that they recommend being part of the daily diet: (1) fruits, (2) grains, (3) vegetables, (4) protein, and (5) dairy.

The "Plate" includes fruits, grains, and vegetables, and suggests that at least three-fifths of a person's caloric intake should be comprised of foods from these three categories.

Incidentally, those categories are foods with high carbohydrate content. Fat is merely mentioned in the context of as oils, which are included as part of food "patterns," instead of being a major food group. Fats from non-aquatic animals, such as beef, pork, and poultry, are not included in the nutritional conversation at all.

However, many recent scientific studies have not only refuted that the exclusion of animal fats from the diet is a good idea. In fact, animal fat is not only an essential component of the human diet, but should be recognized as a major portion of human nutrition, especially when a person is striving to lose weight, and get healthier.

Ketosis

The human body was designed to use fat for energy, and when mostly fat is used for energy, it stores only minimum levels of fat. This results in a lean body, as nature originally designed it, because excessive fat stores are not left inside muscle tissue, "padding" the body.

If one goes on a high-fat diet, and the body is starved of carbohydrates, it will burn fat instead of storing it, and during the metabolic process, it produces "ketones."

A high-carbohydrate diet on the other hand is more likely to result to weight gain because the body can quickly store carbs that are not used for energy and convert it to fat.

Ketones are molecules that are made in the liver from fatty acids, and are generated from the breakdown of fats. Ketones are formed almost as a defensive action by the body: when the body "senses" that there is not enough sugar or glucose to provide for the body's energy needs, it immediately creates an alternative fuel source.

When dietary carbohydrates are suddenly taken away from the diet, more fatty acids are released from fat cells, which leads to fat being metabolized in our liver. This increased burning of fatty acids in the liver eventually causes ketone bodies to be produced, and induces ketosis, a new metabolic state.

Other hormones are likewise affected, and these helps transfer the use of this new fuel, instead of carbohydrates, to body tissues. The majority of calories burned by the human body for energy will now come from this fat breakdown.

In short, ketosis is the process where your body burns fat instead of carbohydrates. When the burned fat comes from fat stores, then your body will be leaner, and the chances of having diseases associated with fat and sugar storage will be minimized, or even eliminated.

Getting to a state of ketosis requires ingesting less than 50 grams of carbohydrates per day, so having a fat counter booklet or app on your phone is the best way to start and continue the diet, in order to measure carbohydrate intake accurately.

Discover Scientifically-Proven "Shortcuts" & "Hacks" to Lose Weight FASTER (With Very Little Effort)

For this month only, you can get Linda's best-selling & most popular book absolutely free – *Weight Loss Secrets You NEED to Know.*

Get Your FREE Copy Here:

TopFitnessAdvice.com/Bonus

Discover scientifically-proven tips to help you lose weight faster and easier than ever before. With this book, readers were able to improve their weight loss results and fitness levels. So, it's highly recommended that you get this book, especially while it's free!

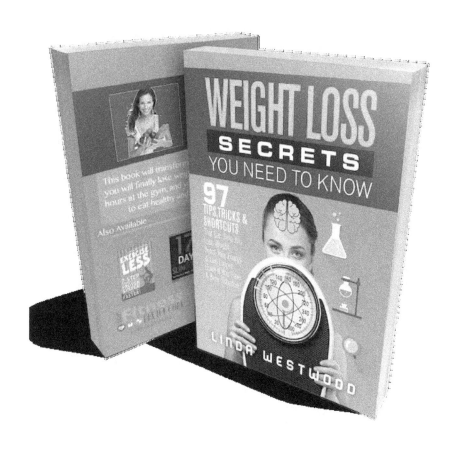

Get Your FREE Copy Here:
TopFitnessAdvice.com/Bonus

Ketosis Mistakes and Misconceptions

It is useful to know what people, even health professionals, say that might end up scaring you off the Ketogenic diet. There are so many myths and misconceptions that have surrounded, and clouded, ketosis and the Ketogenic diet.

Ketosis Myths and Misconceptions

1. **Myth:** Carbohydrates are an essential nutrient for good health.

   The truth: You can get nutrition and energy from protein and fat.

2. **Myth:** Eating a low-carbohydrate diet can lead to vitamin deficiencies, especially Vitamin C, which comes from carbohydrate-rich sugary fruits and vegetables.

   The truth: You can still get vitamins and minerals from some fruits and other food sources

3. **Myth:** Ketogenic diets cause your body to go into a state of ketosis, which is dangerous.

   The truth: Natural ketosis is not harmful to your body. There may be some discomfort at first especially if you're used to a high-carb diet, but it's safe. The misconception is usually brought by lack of understanding of ketosis.

Many people mistake ketosis for ketoacidosis, which is an entirely different condition.

4. **Myth:** Your kidneys will sustain damage from the high protein consumption.

   The truth: With a balanced diet, you should not worry about this at all.

5. **Myth:** A high-fat diet will lead to osteoporosis, because it will cause the body to excrete calcium.

   The truth: You can get calcium from sources other than dairy such as seafood and oysters, beans, and bone broth. You can even get it from dark, leafy greens such as kale and broccoli.

6. **Myth:** Eating fat makes you fat.

   The truth: Dietary fat has little to do with body fat. You don't get fat just by eating fat. You become fat when your calorie intake is way higher than your calorie usage

7. **Myth:** The ketogenic diet leaves out carbohydrates completely.

   The truth: You can have up to 50 grams of carbs every day.

8. **Myth:** Cholesterol from animal fat causes heart disease.

The truth: There is good cholesterol and bad cholesterol. Good cholesterol even reduces your chances of getting certain heart diseases! The ketogenic diet includes food that contains good cholesterol.

Ketosis, of course, means making fat, and to a lesser extent, proteins, a bigger part of the diet. This means relegating carbohydrates to a very minimum intake.

Common Mistakes on Going on The Ketogenic Diet

Because the ketogenic diet is a radical departure from what most people are used to, it is easy to make mistakes. The following are the most common mistakes that can eradicate the benefits of the ketogenic diet, and may even cause harm to your body:

1. **To gain the maximum benefits from the diet, you have to be in a state of ketosis for at least two weeks** - You CANNOT deviate from this, or you will basically need to start from zero again, and allow dangerous carbohydrates to assault your system, and create even more fat.

2. **Eating too much processed fats and proteins** - This is especially true for boxed or TV dinners. While they may have a lot of fat content, there are usually a lot of hidden sugars, and worse, artificial chemicals that can derail your progress.

Just because a boxed or frozen meal is high-fat does not necessarily mean is advantageous for someone who is on a ketogenic diet.

3. **Eating more protein as opposed to fat** - Fat will be your main source of energy, and eating excess protein can actually be harmful, because some of it is converted to sugar.

4. **Being afraid of fat** - In the dietary world, fat is the friend, and we need to forget all the misconceptions about it.

5. **Not getting enough water** - Water is the most important element of any diet, and it sometimes helps to give the body a feeling of "fullness."

Optimal Foods, Safe Foods and Bad Foods for Ketosis

What we are is what we eat, and this is even more important to remember when one is on the ketogenic diet. It is therefore, very important to know what we can, and what we shouldn't eat.

What to Eat

- Animal Meats: Beef, veal, pork, lamb, goat, venison, and other wild game. Organic and grass-fed cuts are the healthiest options.
- Bacon, pork rinds, and sausage: Make sure that there are no added sugars or excess preservatives.
- Poultry: All kinds, and be liberal with the skin and the fat portions. No need to skim them off anymore. Once again, organic and grass-fed cuts are the healthiest options. Eggs, especially the yolks, are highly recommended. Organic eggs or eggs from grass-fed chickens are preferred.
- Fish of all varieties, with "fattier" varieties, such as tuna, salmon, mackerel, and trout.
- Peanut butter, if very low in carbohydrates, and no sugar content.
- Milk, butter, and cheese (watch out for blends! They may have sugars and other dangerous chemicals)
- Avocados and dried, unsweetened coconuts.
- Non-starchy, green, leafy vegetables, such as leafy greens like bok choy, lettuce, Swiss card, radicchio, endives.
- Kale, kohlrabi, and radish.

- Green asparagus, celery stalk, cucumber, bamboo shoots, zucchini, cucumber, and summer squash.
- Broth, especially self-made bone broth, non-sweet pickles, kimchi, sauerkraut, and mustard.
- Almost all herbs and spices (no sweeteners and preservatives) and recipe enhancers such as lime juice, lemon, and their grated skins.
- Whey protein (keep away from those with sugar, chemical additives, and soy additives.)
- Nuts (make sure there are no sugar-based additives), such as Brazil nuts, hazelnuts, pecans, walnuts, sunflower seeds, sesame and pumpkin seeds, pistachios, pine nuts, and peanuts.
- Coconut oil, lard, olive oil.

Foods that you can eat but only in moderation

- Bell peppers, shallots, tomatoes
- All kinds of cabbage, cauliflower, broccoli, fennel, rutabaga, turnips. Brussels sprouts, eggplant.
- Coconut, olives, and rhubarb
- Peppers, tomatoes, and eggplant
- Winter squash, leeks, garlic, onions, and mushrooms
- Most berry varieties, including strawberries, blackberries, cranberries, raspberries, and blueberries.

What Not to Eat

- Almost all forms of alcohol. Most pure rums, though, have zero carbohydrates

- Rice
- Breads, including wheat bread
- Pancakes and waffles
- Syrups and chocolate toppings
- Desserts
- Breakfast cereals
- Most so-called energy bars, including protein bars
- Most energy boost drinks
- Chocolate bars and candies
- Ice cream
- T.V. dinners
- Oils that are processed are generally harmful to the body, and will impede ketogenic progress. These include: margarine, sunflower, cottonseed, safflower, canola, grape seed, soybean, and corn oils.
- Sodas and sugary drinks, and most juice drinks. The basic rule is this: You have to avoid foods and drinks with sugars, carbohydrates, preservatives and chemicals.

I hope that you are enjoying this book so far, and if you could spare 30 seconds, I would greatly appreciate you leaving a review on Amazon.com.

Ketosis' Overwhelming Success

Weight and fat loss are the objectives of an overwhelming majority of people going on the ketogenic diet. Of course, the associated benefits of a slimmer body can also lead to a decrease in "bad" cholesterol levels, blood pressure, and just better overall, heart health.

Other benefits from a ketogenic have been observed (but not necessarily scientifically proven beyond a reasonable doubt):

- Brain health
- Reduction of symptoms of Parkinson's disease
- Cancer
- Reduction of symptoms of Mitochondrial Disorders
- Reduction of symptoms of Amyotrophic Lateral Sclerosis (ALS, or Lou Gehrig's disease)
- Reduction of symptoms of Epilepsy, especially in younger people
- Improved Focus and Mental Clarity
- Increased Energy

But for weight loss, results are often dramatic and long lasting. Consider the following cases:

"Allison" came from a family of binge eaters, and indulged in binge eating herself.

At 230 pounds, she had become desperate, and following the program faithfully, she lost almost 25 pounds after the first month. She managed to stay on track and lost 55 pounds over the nine-month period that she was on the ketogenic diet.

"Tommy" was a morbidly obese diabetic. After going on a high-fat diet, he lost 200 pounds over a period of two years, while hardly even exercising.

As he was losing weight using the ketogenic diet, his own diabetes nurse had been a disbelieving witness. Tommy's cholesterol levels, lipid levels, and blood sugar, just kept improving, while eating the exact opposite of the "official" dietary guide we discussed earlier.

There are also those who take the diet in a somewhat light-hearted manner, but also achieve success.

"Harry" lost over 65 pounds in 5 months in 2015, and didn't even bother to count calories, much less own a carbohydrate counter.

Basically, he ate all the eggs, cheese, meat, and green vegetables he could, while drinking a lot of tea and water. He had moderate success in gaining just a bit of weight during the Christmas season while indulging in sweets, but quickly lost the weight again after getting on a ketogenic diet right after the holidays.

What is a Ketogenic Diet?

The Ketogenic Diet

The keto (or ketogenic) diet is a low carbohydrate – high fat diet that typically consists of 70% fat, 25% protein and 5% carbs, unlike a conventional diet which normally has you eating 20% fat, 30% protein and 50% carbs daily.

This diet can be used for many different purposes. Typically, it's been used for therapeutic reasons to help reduce symptoms like high blood pressure, high sugar levels and high cholesterol but more recently it's become more mainstream and is now being used by athletes and body builders for rapid weight loss and optimizing performance.

Essentially the purpose of the keto diet is to stop your body from burning carbohydrates as its main energy source, and train it to metabolize fat instead as its main source of energy. The goal is to put your body into ketosis by maintaining a high fat low carb diet.

What does it mean to be in ketosis?

When your body reduces that amount of carbohydrates it is used to consuming, it goes into a metabolic state called ketosis.

As you continue to increase your daily fat intake and decrease the amount of carbs you eat, your body starts generating and utilizing substances known as ketone bodies which can be used as energy sources for the brain and muscles in your body.

Benefits of the Ketogenic Diet

As I had already mentioned a bit earlier the Ketogenic diet is used by various groups of people for many different reasons. There are medical benefits to following a ketogenic diet such as treatment for diabetes, epilepsy, cancer, heart disease and more.

Outside of medical benefits, here are some of the more mainstream and popular reasons why more people are starting to use the Ketogenic Diet:

- **Helps you lose weight fast**

    Having a low carb diet is actually proven to be one of the fastest ways you can go about losing weight. It is actually even more effective for weight loss than someone who's on a low-fats diet. This is because a low carbs diet actually helps to get rid of the excess water from your body, and as your insulin levels lower your kidneys start to shed excess sodium which leads to rapid weight loss.

- **Kills your appetite**

    Studies have shown that when people cut carbs and start to intake foods that are high in protein, their appetite actually goes down and they end up consuming fewer calories.

- **Reduces blood sugar and insulin levels**

    When we consume carbohydrates, the food breaks down into simple sugars in our bodies which raises our blood sugar levels. When our blood sugar level rises, our bodies insulin levels rise in order to minimize the spike in sugar levels to prevent it from harming us. Therefore, if you reduce the amount of carbs you consume, you can significantly reduce your blood sugar and insulin levels. The Keto diet is actually a very good solution for diabetics.

- **Blood pressure goes down**

    You can reduce the risk of many common health complications like kidney failures, heart diseases and many others by reducing your blood pressure. Consuming less carbs is actually one of the most effective ways of doing this.

- **Good cholesterol goes up**

    I'm sure we've all heard that a high cholesterol can lead to a heart attack, but did you know that there's good and bad cholesterols? The bad cholesterol is known has Low Density Lipoprotein (LDL). Too much LDL floating around in your bloodstream is a bad thing which can lead to you having a heart attack. When you reduce the amount of the carbs in your diet, your LDL changes to what's called large LDL which is benign.

As you can see, there are definitely a lot of upsides to the Keto diet. Unlike many diets you might heard of, the ketogenic diet is not a fad diet. There are many lifelong benefits to it and it is actually not as restrictive as you might think. People that follow the Keto diet can still enjoy most foods while maintaining a realistic lifestyle.

The Mediterranean-keto fused recipes in this book are crafted so that you get to enjoy great tasting meals while reaping the multitudes of benefits from following a cleaner diet that will transform your body from within.

Enjoying this book?

Check out my other best sellers!

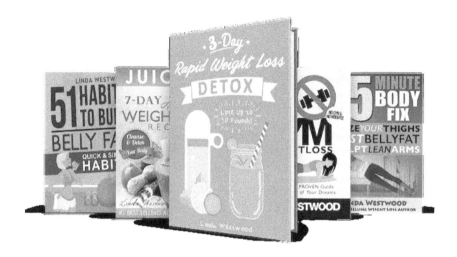

Get your next book on sale here:

TopFitnessAdvice.com/go/books

Breakfast Recipes

Keto Cereal

Star your day with this cereal! For more flavor, try toasting the coconut flakes ahead of time, or mix them together with stevia and cinnamon in a zip lock bag. During a busy day, all you need to do is put all of the ingredients together in a bowl. Instant cereal! You can also store this mix for later as a handy snack option.

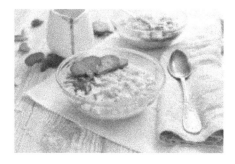

Prep Time: 5 minutes
Cook Time: 5 minutes

Serving Size: 257 g
Serves: 1
Calories: 593
Total Fat: 121 g
Saturated Fat: 17.8 g
Trans Fat: 0 g
Protein: 2.7 g
Net Carbs: 2.8 g
Total Carbs: 14 g
Dietary Fibre: 6.8 g

Sugars: 6.7 g
Cholesterol: 0 mg
Sodium: 13 mg
Potassium: 314 mg
Vitamin A: 0%
Vitamin C: 65%
Calcium: 1%
Iron: 48%

Ingredients

- 1 package of flaked coconut
- Ground cinnamon
- Stevia
- Almond milk
- A few medium sized strawberries
- Parchment paper and coconut oil

Directions

1. Preheat oven to 350 degrees. Line a cookie sheet with parchment paper and cover with coconut oil. Pour coconut flakes onto the cookie sheet.

2. Cook in oven for five minutes. Shuffle the flakes around and keep cooking until they are light brown and toasted. Sprinkle lightly with cinnamon.

3. Pour ½ cup of the coconut chips into a bowl. Pour the unsweetened almond milk over them. Slice up strawberries for garnish and eat.

Coconut Pancakes

These high-fat pancakes are insanely delicious. They are pillowy, fluffy, super coconutty, tender, perfectly sweet, healthy, and easy to make. I love sprinkling the top with toasted coconut flake for a slightly crunchy version. You can even make these ahead of time, freeze them for up to 2 days, and then reheat them in the microwave.

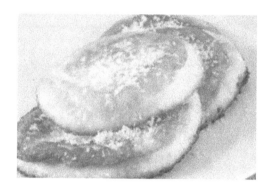

Prep Time: 8 minutes
Cook Time: 6 minutes

Serving Size: 157 g
Serves: 1 (2 pieces 8-inch pancakes)
Calories: 326
Total Fat: 26 g
Saturated Fat: 14.3 g
Trans Fat: 0 g
Protein: 17.1g
Net Carbs: 1.6 g
Total Carbs: 2.5 g
Dietary Fibre: 0.9 g
Sugars: 1.7 g

Cholesterol: 522 mg
Sodium: 424 mg
Potassium: 216 mg
Vitamin A: 0%
Vitamin C: 65%
Calcium: 1%
Iron: 48%

Ingredients

- 3 eggs
- 2 tablespoons coconut flour
- 1 tablespoon butter
- Kosher salt

Directions

1. In mixing bowl, beat the eggs, coconut flour, a pinch of salt until well combined.

2. In a non-stick skillet over medium heat, melt 1/2 tablespoon of the butter.

3. Pour half of the batter mixture. Cook for about 2, flip, and then cook for about 1 minute more or until the pancake is cooked through. Cook the remaining batter with the remaining 1/2 tablespoon butter. Serve topped with leftover meat or avocado slices, if desired.

Spicy Keto Omelet

This healthy and quick breakfast idea came to me when I had leftover shrimp from the night before. They looked kind of lonely sitting on their own, so I thought they'd love a little bit of company. I gathered up what I had in the pantry and the fridge, and came up with this very pleasing omelet. I love spicy food so I made my version hotter with more cayenne.

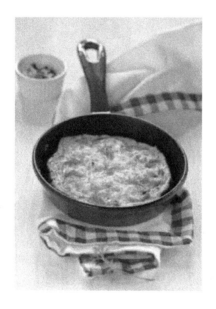

Prep Time: 10 minutes
Cook Time: 5 minutes

Serving Size: 239 g
Serves: 4
Calories: 248
Total Fat: 20.6 g
Saturated Fat: 16.8 g
Trans Fat: 0 g

Protein: 10.2 g
Net Carbs: 5.7 g
Total Carbs: 8.1 g
Dietary Fibre: 2.4 g
Sugars: 4.6 g
Cholesterol: 81 mg
Sodium: 96 mg
Potassium: 515 mg
Vitamin A: 50%
Vitamin C: 38%
Calcium: 5%
Iron: 6%

Ingredients

- 10 large shrimps
- 30 ml of almond milk
- Six eggs (4-5 are egg whites and 1 is the egg yolk)
- 4 grape tomatoes
- 5 tablespoons coconut oil
- 1/8 pound of spinach
- 1 small onion
- 1 sprig of parsley
- ¼ teaspoon of cayenne pepper

Directions

1. Chop the veggies. Beat the egg whites, egg yolk and almond milk together.

2. Coat a small frying pan with coconut oil. Sauté the veggies until they are soft. Remove the veggies and pour in the eggs.

3. When the eggs are firm, place ½ the veggies on ½ the egg mixtures. Fold the egg mixture over the top. Place the remaining veggies on the top of the omelet. Eat and enjoy!

Creamy Cheesy Asparagus Frittata

This is combining everything you love in a skillet and then baking them into flavorful, cheesy, fluffy perfection. This breakfast-dinner dish or briner is both delicious and easy to make. Not only does this taste great, your house will also smell amazing when the frittata is cooked.

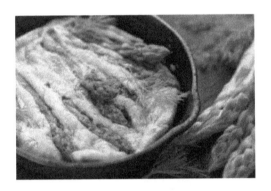

Prep Time: 15 minutes
Cook Time: 30 minutes

Serving Size: 159 g
Serves: 8
Calories: 258
Total Fat: 20.4 g
Saturated Fat: 9.6 g
Trans Fat: 0 g
Protein: 13 g
Net Carbs: 3.2 g
Total Carbs: 4.5 g
Dietary Fibre: 1.3 g
Sugars: 1.9 g
Cholesterol: 222 mg

Sodium: 334 mg
Potassium: 218 mg
Vitamin A: 21%
Vitamin C: 6%
Calcium: 20%
Iron: 13%

Ingredients

- 8 large eggs
- pound asparagus, choose slender stalks if available, ends trimmed
- 1/2 cup Parmesan cheese, grated, divided
- 1 cup Swiss cheese, shredded
- 4 tablespoons butter
- 1/4 cup heavy cream
- 1/2 teaspoon salt
- 1/2 teaspoon dried thyme
- 1/2 small onion
- 1/2 cup dry white wine
- 2 tablespoons-worth nonstick cooking spray, for greasing

Directions

1. Lay the asparagus stalks on a cutting board. Cut each stalk into 1/2 inches. Grease a heavy oven-safe skillet well with cooking spray. Place over medium-low heat. Melt the butter. Put the onion. Sauté until soft and translucent.

2. Add the asparagus. Sauté for 1–2 minutes or until the stalks turn brighter green.

3. In a mixing bowl, whisk the remaining ingredients together. Pour into the skillet. Stir around until the onions and the asparagus are distributed evenly.

4. Adjust the heat to low. Cover the skillet. Cook for about 15–20 minutes. Check. If the frittata is still runny, cook for additional 5–10 minutes.

5. When the frittata is just a little runny, transfer the skillet into the oven about 6 inches from the heat. Broil for until the top is just golden. Cut into wedges. Serve.

Feta Cheese and Pesto Sauce Omelet with Grilled Vegetable

This is a great way to give leftover vegetables a new look and a different taste. What I like to do is place the omelet in a deep plate, top it with the heated grilled vegetables, drizzle pesto sauce all over the veggies, and then sprinkle it with the cheese and sea salt. It's a new dish that barely resembles what you ate just last night!

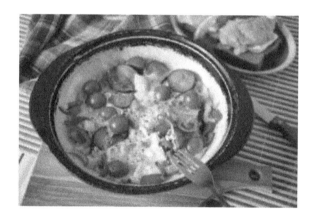

Prep Time: 10 minutes
Cook Time: 10 minutes

Serving Size: 143 g
Serves: 1
Calories: 406
Total Fat: 37.8 g
Saturated Fat: 8.6 g
Trans Fat: 0 g
Protein: 15.4 g
Net Carbs: 2.6 g
Total Carbs: 3.1 g

Dietary Fibre: 0.5 g
Sugars: 0 g
Cholesterol: 343 mg
Sodium: 418 mg
Potassium: 124 mg
Vitamin A: 1%
Vitamin C: 0%
Calcium: 19%
Iron: 10%

Ingredients

- 1 tablespoon olive oil or butter
- 2 eggs, well beaten
- 2 tablespoons pesto sauce
- 1 tablespoon feta cheese
- Optional: 1 1/2 cups leftover grilled vegetables, chopped
- For taste: Sea salt

Directions

1. If using vegetables, pour vegetables in a small pot, cover, and heat over medium-low heat. When sufficiently heated, set aside. Over medium heat, heat the oil in a small skillet.

2. In a bowl, whisk the eggs until well beaten. Pour the beaten eggs into the skillet. Cook for about 2–3 minutes or until the center and sides of the eggs are firm. Carefully flip. Cook for an additional 10–20 seconds.

3. When cooked, transfer to a plate. Stuff the vegetables. Serve with feta cheese, pesto sauce, and a sprinkle of sea salt.

Once again, thank you for reading this book, and I hope you're getting a lot of valuable information. I would greatly appreciate it if you could take 30 seconds to leave me a review for this book on Amazon.com.

Breakfast Green Eggs

Sam-I-Am would certainly love this version of green eggs. It's definitely a journey of a whimsically delicious breakfast in the world of Dr. Seuss. Top this dish with a spoonful or two of Keto Mexican Guacamole and low-carb salsa, and your tastes buds will thank you.

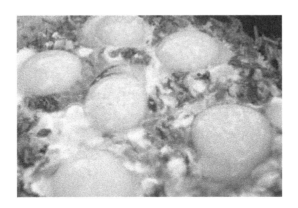

Prep Time: 5 minutes
Cook Time: 15 minutes

Serving Size: 187 g
Serves: 1
Calories: 351
Total Fat: 32 g
Saturated Fat: 17.4 g
Trans Fat: 0 g
Protein: 13.3 g
Net Carbs: 3.2 g
Total Carbs: 4.6 g
Dietary Fibre: 1.4 g
Sugars: 0 g
Cholesterol: 388 mg

Sodium: 490 mg
Potassium: 494 mg
Vitamin A: 138%
Vitamin C: 29%
Calcium: 12%
Iron: 19%

Ingredients

- 2 eggs
- 2 cups frozen spinach
- 1 small shallot
- 2 tablespoons butter
- Salt
- Black pepper

Directions

1. Heat up the spinach in the microwave for about 1 minute to defrost.

2. While the spinach is heating up, mince shallot. In a small cast iron skillet over medium heat, heat the butter. Put the shallot in and sauté.

3. Beat the eggs with the salt and pepper. Squeeze out the liquid from the spinach. Add into the egg mix. Stir to combine. Pour into the skillet, making sure the shallots are distributed.

4. Lower the heat to medium-low. Cook until the frittata is set, flip, and continue cooking until thoroughly cooked. Serve with guacamole and salsa, if desired.

Baked Eggs and Avocado

Baking eggs and avocado together is a great way of filling your day with the heart-healthy fat omega 3. The baked eggs and bacon come out warm and creamy. Topped with delicious crispy salty bacon crumbs, this makes for a scrumptious morning meal!

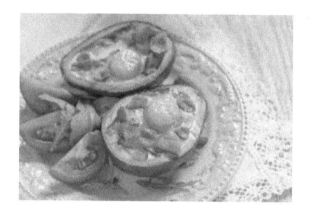

Prep Time: 10 minutes
Cook Time: 15 minutes

Serving Size: 157 g
Serves: 2
Calories: 361
Total Fat: 31.2 g
Saturated Fat: 7.9 g
Trans Fat: 0 g
Protein: 13.6 g
Net Carbs: 5.9 g
Total Carbs: 6.7 g
Dietary Fibre: 0.8 g
Sugars: 0.8 g

Cholesterol: 159 mg
Sodium: 497 mg
Potassium: 644 mg
Vitamin A: 7%
Vitamin C: 17%
Calcium: 3%
Iron: 9%

Ingredients

- 1 avocado; cut in half and pit
- 2 slices bacon, cooked and crumbled
- 2 small eggs

To season

- Chives
- Parsley
- Sea salt
- Pepper

Directions

1. Preheat oven to 425F (220C). Carefully crack the eggs into a bowl, making sure the yolks remain intact.

2. Arrange the avocado halves in a baking dish. Rest them along the edge so they will not tip over. Gently and carefully, spoon 1 egg yolk into an avocado pit.

3. Spoon egg white into the avocado until the pit is full. Repeat the process for the other avocado half. Season each filled avocado pit with parsley, chives, salt, and pepper.

4. Carefully place the baking dish in the oven; bake for about 15 minutes or until the eggs are cooked. Sprinkle crumbled bacon over the cooked avocado and eggs.

Eggs Benedict Sandwich

Missing bread? Then make your own cream cheese Oopsie rolls (see recipe below). These no carb and no flour rolls are good substitutes for real breads and are easy to whip up. Topped with Canadian bacon, poached egg, and hollandaise sauce, this sandwich is a perfect breakfast. This version is a high fat, high-protein, rich in vitamins and minerals meal that is exactly what you need to start the day right.

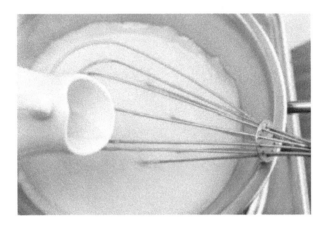

Prep Time: 10 minutes
Cook Time: 10 minutes

Serving Size: 153 g
Serves: 4
Calories: 316
Total Fat: 25.7 g
Saturated Fat: 12.3 g
Trans Fat: 0 g
Protein: 19.2 g
Net Carbs: 2.2 g
Total Carbs: 2.2 g

Dietary Fibre: 0 g
Sugars: 0.8 g
Cholesterol: 461 mg
Sodium: 737 mg
Potassium: 267 mg
Vitamin A: 21%
Vitamin C: 1%
Calcium: 8%
Iron: 12%

Ingredients

- 4 eggs
- 1 tablespoon vinegar
- 1 tsp. chives
- 4 Oopsie rolls
- 4 slices Canadian back bacon

Hollandaise Sauce

- 2 egg yolks
- 2 tablespoons butter
- 2 pinches paprika
- 1 tsp lemon juice
- a pinch of salt

Directions

1. Make a quick hollandaise sauce. Separate 2 eggs and whisk the yolks in a glass bowl until they've doubled in

volume. Add a splash of lemon juice. Boil a pot of water and melt butter. Add to the sauce to emulsify.

2. Use a double boiler and whisk the egg yolks rapidly. They become thicker the more you whisk, but do not cook the too much or they will become scrambled eggs. Hollandaise Sauce should be spoonable.

3. Poach your eggs in a pot of water. Use about 3 inches of water. Once the water comes to a boil, reduce it to simmer and add salt and white vinegar. Create a whirlpool in the water with a wooden spoon – stir the water around a few times in one direction.

4. Crack an egg into a teacup and gently lower it into the whirlpool you have created. Lower the egg in the water; don't drop the egg in. Cook the egg for about 2-4 minutes. The eggs need to be runny.

5. Lift the egg out with a spatula and rest it on a paper towel. Fry up the Canadian bacon. Top 4 Oopsie rolls with the Canadian bacon and place poached egg on top. Spoon hollandaise sauce onto each poached egg, add salt and pepper, and enjoy!

Keto Lemon-Poppy Seed Muffins

These muffins are fast and easy to make. They are also great to store and are freezable as well. Perfect when you are in a hurry during a busy weekday.

Heat a piece in the microwave for about 15-20 seconds, slice in half, and dab a slice of butter between the slices for extra fat. You can also enjoy them as a snack topped with whipped cream cheese frosting.

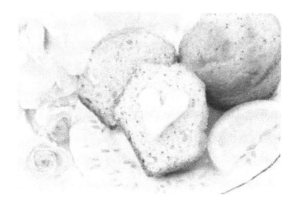

Prep Time: 15 minutes
Cook Time: 20 minutes

Serving Size: 44 g
Serves: 12
Calories: 120
Total Fat: 10.4 g
Saturated Fat: 3.8 g
Trans Fat: 0 g
Protein: 3.8 g
Net Carbs: 1.1 g
Total Carbs: 3.7 g

Dietary Fibre: 1.8 g
Sugars: 0.9 g
Cholesterol: 60 mg
Sodium: 48 mg
Potassium: 154 mg
Vitamin A: 4%
Vitamin C: 12%
Calcium: 7%
Iron: 8%

Ingredients

- 3/4 cup almond flour
- 1/4 cup flaxseed meal
- 1/3 cup Erythritol
- 1 teaspoon baking powder
- 2 tablespoon poppy seeds
- 1/4 cup melted butter
- 1/4 cup heavy cream
- 3 large eggs
- Zest of 2 lemons
- 3 tablespoons lemon juice
- 1 teaspoon vanilla extract

Directions

1. Preheat oven to 350F. Combine almond flour, flaxseed meal, Erythritol and poppy seeds. Stir in melted butter, eggs, and heavy cream. Mix until no lumps are in the batter.

2. Add in baking powder, vanilla extract, lemon zest, and lemon juice. Mix thoroughly. Pour batter into baking cups. Bake for 18-20 minutes or until slightly browned.

3. Remove from the oven and cool for about 10 minutes. Makes a total of 12 Keto Lemon Poppy Seed Muffins

Almond Butter Pancakes

These pancakes are absolutely grain-free. This breakfast closely resembles a stack of real pancakes, both in flavor and texture. Most will not believe they are flour-less. For added flavor, top with sugar-free maple syrup.

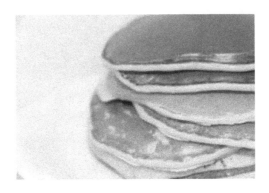

Prep Time: 5 minutes
Cook Time: 30 minutes

Serving Size: 115 g
Serves: 4
Calories: 496
Total Fat: 46.6 g
Saturated Fat: 17.2 g
Trans Fat: 0 g
Protein: 14.8 g
Net Carbs: 3 g
Total Carbs: 9.7 g
Dietary Fibre: 1.8 g
Sugars: 0 g
Cholesterol: 150 mg
Sodium: 131 mg

Potassium: 601 mg
Vitamin A: 6%
Vitamin C: 1%
Calcium: 23%
Iron: 14%

Ingredients

- 3/4 cup almond butter
- 3 large eggs
- 2 tablespoons water
- 1/8 teaspoon salt
- 1/4 cup heavy cream
- 1/4 cup coconut oil
- 1 1/2 teaspoons baking powder

Directions

1. Over medium heat, heat a heavy, large non-stick skillet or a girdle. Put all of the ingredients into a blender. Blend until you have a smooth batter.

2. Grease the skillet or girdle with 1 tablespoon coconut oil. Pour batter into the skillet or girdle. Cook until the bottom side is browned. Flip and continue cooking until thoroughly cooked.

Cheesy Ham Stromboli

This recipe is great finger food that can also be made ahead of time. Cut the Stromboli into 4 large pieces or into 8 small slices and bake to cheesy and crispy perfection. Serve with roasted broccoli and butter for a delicious breakfast.

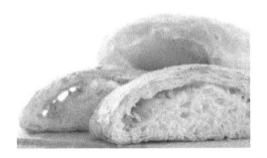

Prep Time: 20 minutes
Cook Time: 20 minutes

Serving Size: 155 g
Serves: 4
Calories: 488
Total Fat: 38.6 g
Saturated Fat: 22.3 g
Trans Fat: 0 g
Protein: 26.8 g
Net Carbs: 6.2 g
Total Carbs: 11.9 g
Dietary Fibre: 5.7 g
Sugars: 3.4 g
Cholesterol: 108 mg
Sodium: 762 mg
Potassium: 366 mg

Vitamin A: 11%
Vitamin C: 6%
Calcium: 48%
Iron: 37%

Ingredients

- 4 ounces ham
- 4 tablespoons almond flour
- 3 tablespoons coconut flour
- 3 1/2 ounces cheddar cheese
- 1 1/4 cups mozzarella cheese, shredded
- 1 large egg
- 1 teaspoon Italian seasoning
- Salt and pepper, to taste

Directions

1. Preheat the oven to 400F. In a mixing bowl, combine the coconut flour, the almond flour, and the rest of the seasoning. In a microwave, melt the mozzarella cheese. Heat for about 1 minute, then in 10 seconds interval afterwards, stirring occasionally. You can also melt it in a toaster oven for about 10 minutes.

2. When the mozzarella cheese has melted, allow to cool down for a little bit. Add it into the flour mixture. Add in the egg. Combine everything until the mixture becomes a moist dough. Transfer into a flat surface lined with parchment paper.

3. Place a second sheet of parchment paper over the dough. With a rolling pin or your hand, flatten the dough. With a knife or a pizza cutter, cut diagonal lines from the dough edges towards the center, leaving a row of uncut dough, about 4 inches wide.

4. On the uncut surface of the dough, lay the ham and then cheddar. Layer alternately. One section of the cut dough at a time, lay it over the top of the filling, covering it; bake for about 15–20 minutes or until it has turned to a golden brown. Slice and serve.

Crunchy Eggplant

Made with gluten-free, low carb ingredients, the crispy eggplant makes for a satisfying ketogenic meal. This recipe is also great as a snack or side dish. Coated with pork rind crumbs, the eggplant is deliciously flavorful with a nice crispy, cheesy texture.

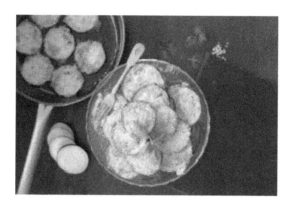

Prep Time: 30 minutes
Cook Time: 20-30 minutes

Serving Size: 244 g
Serves: 4
Calories: 528
Total Fat: 44.9 g
Saturated Fat: 19.9 g
Trans Fat: 0 g
Protein: 22.7 g
Net Carbs: 4.2 g
Total Carbs: 10.3 g
Dietary Fibre: 6.1 g
Sugars: 5.1 g
Cholesterol: 116 mg

Sodium: 683 mg
Potassium: 381 mg
Vitamin A: 1%
Vitamin C: 6%
Calcium: 2%
Iron: 14%

Ingredients

- 1 cup pork rind crumbs
- 1 large egg
- 1 medium-size globe eggplant
- 1/2 cup bacon grease, or more as needed
- 1/4 cup coconut flour
- 2 teaspoons water
- Salt

Directions

1. Cut the eggplant into about 1/4-inch slices. Lightly sprinkle both sides of the slices with salt. Allow to sit for about 20-30 minutes.

2. Put the coconut flour on a plate. Beat the eggs and water together. Pour in a concave plate. On another plate, put the pork rind crumbs. Arrange in that order.

3. Heat the bacon grease in a heavy skillet over medium heat. Pat dry the eggplant slices. Dredge an eggplant in the coconut flour, then coat it with the egg wash, and then coat with the pork rind crumbs.

4. Fry the eggplant in hot grease until both sides are crisp and brown. Add more grease as needed. Serve hot topped with fried eggs.

Butternut Squash Porridge

This is a dairy-free and gluten-free recipe. Butternut squash is pumpkin's cousin. However, it has a higher beta-carotene level. It is also packed with B vitamins and minerals.

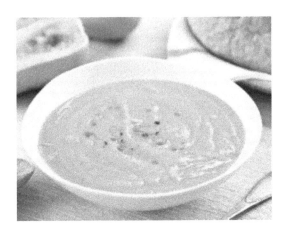

Prep Time: 10 minutes
Cook Time: 50 minutes

Serving Size: 286 g
Serves: 3
Calories: 430
Total Fat: 36.2 g
Saturated Fat: 22.9 g
Trans Fat: 0 g
Protein: 3.5 g
Net Carbs: 23.5 g
Total Carbs: 29.0 g
Dietary Fibre: 5.5 g
Sugars: 5.8 g
Cholesterol: 76 mg
Sodium: 13 mg

Potassium: 891 mg
Vitamin A: 514%
Vitamin C: 83%
Calcium: 12%
Iron: 12%

Ingredients

- 1/4 cup (or more to taste) coconut milk
- 1/2 teaspoon ground cinnamon
- 1 tablespoon walnuts, chopped
- 1 butternut squash; cut in half and seed
- Water as needed
- 7 tablespoons ghee

Directions

1. Preheat oven to 350F (175C). With the cut-side up, place the butternut squash halves into a baking dish. Fill the dish with 1/4-inch water. Place in oven. Bake for about 50–60 minutes, until softened. Cool the cooked butter squash.

2. Scoop the cooked squash into a bowl. Mash using a potato masher or fork until smooth. Add ghee; stir to combine well. Pour the coconut milk and add the cinnamon into the bowl of mashed squash. Stir. Top with walnuts.

Lunch Recipes

Lettuce Wrapped Egg Salad Sandwich

This high-fat, high protein, low-carb meal is great to take to work. You can enjoy this as a snack or you can serve this as a barbecue side dish.

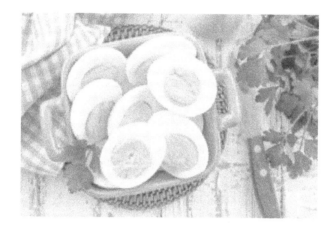

Prep Time: 10 minutes
Cook Time: 0 minutes

Serving Size: 99 g
Serves: 4
Calories: 371
Total Fat: 28.4 g
Saturated Fat: 9 g
Trans Fat: 0 g
Protein: 25.4 g
Net Carbs: 2.1 g
Total Carbs: 2.1 g
Dietary Fibre: 0 g

Sugars: 0.6g
Cholesterol: 186 mg
Sodium: 1551 mg
Potassium: 373 mg
Vitamin A: 4%
Vitamin C: 1%
Calcium: 3%
Iron: 8%

Ingredients

- 2 lettuce leaves
- 3 eggs
- 6 cooked bacon
- 1 tablespoon mayonnaise
- 1 teaspoon Dijon mustard
- 1 teaspoon lemon juice
- ¼ teaspoon salt

Directions

1. Cook the eggs gently in a medium saucepan. Bring to a boil for ten minutes. Remove from heat and cool. Peel the eggs under cold running water.

2. Add the eggs to a food processor and pulse until chopped. Stir in the mayonnaise, mustard, lemon juice, and salt and pepper. Taste and adjust as necessary. Serve with lettuce leaves and bacon for wrapping, if desired.

Crab Louie

This recipe is also known as Crab Louis or the King of Salads and the original version dates as far as in the early 1900s and is believed to have originated on the West Coast of America. The more crab meat, the better!

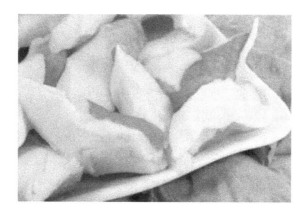

Prep Time: 10 minutes
Cook Time: 0 minutes

Serving Size: 424 g
Serves: 4
Calories: 461
Total Fat: 41.2 g
Saturated Fat: 6.7 g;
Trans Fat: 0 g
Protein: 22.4 g
Net Carbs: 13.7 g
Total Carbs: 18 g
Dietary Fibre: 4.3 g
Sugars: 6.5 g
Cholesterol: 218 mg

Sodium: 918 mg
Potassium: 562 mg
Vitamin A: 42%
Vitamin C: 32%
Calcium: 36%
Iron: 40%

Ingredients

- 6 cups lettuce leaves or salad greens
- 4 eggs, hard-boiled, sliced into halves
- 1/4 cup minced chives
- 1/2 cup of your favorite Louisiana Rémoulade dressing
- 3/4-pound lump crab meat, cooked
- 1 pound asparagus, trimmed
- 1 cup cherry tomatoes
- 6 tablespoons vegetable oil

Directions

1. In a pot of boiling salted water, blanch the asparagus for about 1 minute. Immediately transfer blanched asparagus into a bowl of cold water. When the asparagus are cool, drain the water and toss with the vegetable oil.

2. Divide the lettuce into 4 plates. Arrange the crab meat, the asparagus, tomatoes, and hard-boiled eggs into the 4 plates. Garnish with chives. Serve with the rémoulade on the side.

Others who are considering purchasing this book would love to know what you think. If you could spare a few seconds, they would greatly appreciate reading an honest review from you. Simply visit the page on Amazon.com.

Lettuce Wrapped Tuna-Avocado

Simple yet flavorful tuna and avocado salad is a healthy, light lunch recipe that can also be enjoyed as an appetizer or snack.

Here's a fun fact: not only are lettuce leaves a healthier option than bread, these leaves keep teeth white and the iron in lettuce helps form an acid-resistant barrier in your mouth, which protects your enamel from damage!

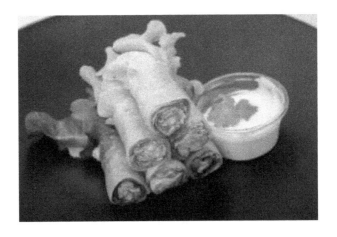

Prep Time: 15 minutes
Cook Time: 0 minutes

Serving Size: 153 g (per wrap)
Serves: 1
Calories: 285
Total Fat: 23.4 g
Saturated Fat: 10.4 g
Trans Fat: 0 g
Protein: 14.4 g
Net Carbs: 8.4 g
Total Carbs: 7.8 g

Dietary Fibre: 4.2 g
Sugars: 0.9 g
Cholesterol: 52 mg
Sodium: 136 mg
Potassium: 489 mg
Vitamin A: 12%
Vitamin C: 22%
Calcium: 2%
Iron: 4%

Ingredients

- 2 butter lettuce leaves
- 1/2 medium avocado
- 1/2 lime
- 1/2 jalapeño, diced small
- 1 scallion, thinly sliced
- 4 ounces wild albacore tuna, canned in water, drained
- 2 tablespoons ghee
- Black pepper, freshly ground
- Kosher salt

Directions

1. Put the tuna in a medium sized bowl. With a fork, gently break the fish into pieces. Add in the scallions and the jalapeño. Toss well. Add in the ghee, salt, and pepper. Squeeze a spritz of lime. Mix together.

2. In a separate bowl, mash half an avocado with salt, pepper, and the rest of the lime juice. Add into the tuna

mixture. Stir to combine. Divide the tuna salad mixture into 2 portions. Place into the lettuce leaves. Wrap and eat up.

Keto Taco Salad

This easy version of the Mexican taco is a salad that may become your favorite go to recipe. With sour cream and salsa on the side, you can pack the taco mixture easily and take it with you for lunch.

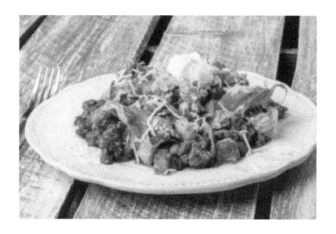

Prep Time: 10 minutes
Cook Time: 10 minutes

Serving Size: 202 g
Serves: 6
Calories: 511
Total Fat: 40.5 g
Saturated Fat: 16.9 g
Trans Fat: 0 g
Protein: 32.2 g
Net Carbs: 3.9 g
Total Carbs: 4.5 g
Dietary Fibre: 0.6 g
Sugars: 1.3 g
Cholesterol: 112 mg

Sodium: 534 mg
Potassium: 510 mg
Vitamin A: 14%
Vitamin C: 2%
Calcium: 35%
Iron: 9%

Ingredients

- 16 ounce. ground pork
- 9 ounce. cheddar cheese, shredded
- 6 tsp McCormick taco seasoning
- 8 tablespoon vegetable oil
- 12 tablespoon sour cream
- 12 tablespoon salsa
- 6 romaine leaves
- Cayenne pepper to taste

Directions

1. Brown the pork in a skillet with the oil. Once the meat is browned, add taco seasoning and any additional spices. Cook until the taco seasoning is incorporated.

2. Let cool, and then distribute into 6 containers. Add cheese to each container. Add sour cream and salsa to a prep bowl and plastic wrap it. Add Romaine lettuce to the container.

Cheesy Bacon Wrapped Hot Dogs

Here is another very simple yet super delicious low carb lunch that you can eat for dinner, too! These dogs are very rich, savory, and fatty.

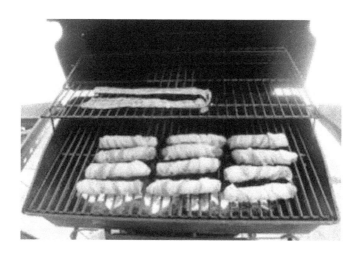

Prep Time: 10 minutes
Cook Time: 20 minutes

Serving Size: 105 g
Makes: 8
Calories: 379
Total Fat: 30.5 g
Saturated Fat: 16.1 g
Trans Fat: 0 g
Protein: 23.1 g
Net Carbs: 1.9 g
Total Carbs: 1.9 g
Dietary Fibre: 0 g
Sugars: 0.7 g
Cholesterol: 91 mg

Sodium: 912 mg
Potassium: 205 mg
Vitamin A: 12%
Vitamin C: 2%
Calcium: 41%
Iron: 2%

Ingredients

- 8 sausage links
- 8 strips bacon
- 16 slices pepper jack cheese
- Black pepper
- Garlic powder
- Onion powder
- Paprika

Directions

1. Cook sausage links on a grill until they're just almost done. Let them cool. Cut a slit in the middle of the sausage links. Place 2 slices of cheese into the middle of each dog.

2. Wrap each dog tightly in bacon. Secure with wet toothpicks to make sure the bacon doesn't shrivel and open up the dog.

3. Sprinkle with your spices and grill on your BBQ grill until the bacon is crispy (about 15–20 minutes). Flip halfway through. Place on plate with low-carb sides and eat away!

Tuna Burgers

These patties make for easy and quick weekday lunch meals. Adding olive oil to the mixture makes sure that they do not get dry. Tuna contains omega 3 fatty acids and is a good way to get a dose of heart-healthy oil.

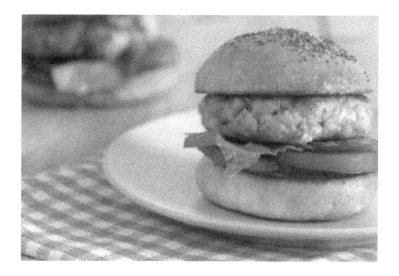

Prep Time: 20 minutes
Cook Time: 10 minutes

Serving Size: 203 g
Makes: 4
Calories: 544
Total Fat: 37.4 g
Saturated Fat: 6.9 g
Trans Fat: 0 g
Protein: 37.4 g
Net Carbs: 7.1 g
Total Carbs: 3.8 g
Dietary Fibre: 1.6 g

Sugars: 1.1 g
Cholesterol: 158 mg
Sodium: 556 mg
Potassium: 545 mg
Vitamin A: 6%
Vitamin C: 6%
Calcium: 6%
Iron: 11%

Ingredients

- 1 tablespoon ginger root, grated
- 1/2 cup almond meal
- 1/4 cup cilantro, chopped
- 2 cans (8-ounce) tuna; drain
- 2 tablespoons lemon juice
- 4 tablespoons olive oil
- 2 tablespoons soy sauce
- 3 eggs
- kosher salt and ground black pepper to taste
- For frying: 3 tablespoons olive oil

Directions

1. Except for the olive oil for frying, mix all the ingredients by hand or using a food processor until the ingredients are well incorporated and the mix becomes firm in consistency. Divide the mix into four equal portions and form into patties.

2. In a skillet or grill pan, heat the 1 tablespoon of olive oil over medium heat. Cook the tuna burgers for about five minutes each side or until the patties and set and the sides are browned. Enjoy with your favorite paleo-friendly burger bun with avocado, lettuce, and tomato.

Nutty Vegetable Patties

These delicious low carb, vegetable burgers are addictive. The seeds give the patties fantastic texture and crunch with a nutty taste. They are gluten-free with only veggies as ingredients. Enjoy them between your favorite low carb burger bun with avocado, lettuce, and tomato.

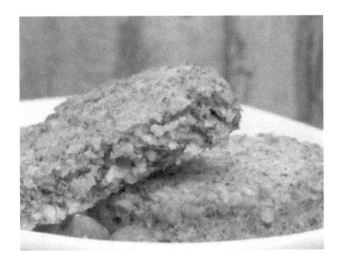

Prep Time: 15 minutes
Cook Time: 15 minutes

Serving Size: 76 g
Makes: 4
Calories: 196
Total Fat: 17.2 g
Saturated Fat: 1.6 g
Trans Fat: 0 g
Protein: 6.5 g
Net Carbs: 7.1 g
Total Carbs: 7.7 g

Dietary Fibre: 3.2 g
Sugars: 1.5 g
Cholesterol: 0 mg
Sodium: 300 mg
Potassium: 303 mg
Vitamin A: 51%
Vitamin C: 35%
Calcium: 5%
Iron: 7%

Ingredients

- 2/3 cup mashed butternut squash, cut into 1/2-inch cubes for steaming
- 1/2 cup cauliflower, chopped
- 1/2 cup broccoli, chopped
- 1/8 teaspoon ground black pepper
- 1/4 teaspoon ground cumin
- 1/4 cup sunflower seed kernels, raw
- 1/4 cup almonds, raw
- 1/2 teaspoon salt
- 1/2 cup walnuts, raw
- 1 tablespoon vegetable oil

Directions

1. Into a saucepan, place a steamer insert. Fill the saucepan with water just below the bottom of the steamer. Bring the water to a boil. Add the butternut squash cubes. Steam for about 7–10 minutes or until tender. Transfer

the cooked squash into a bowl and then mash. Measure 1/2 cup of mashed butternut squash, reserve.

2. Return the steamer insert into the saucepan. Refill with water just below the bottom of the steamer. Bring water to boil. Add in the broccoli and the cauliflower. Cover and steam for about 2-6 minutes until tender. When cooked, transfer the cauliflower into a bowl. Set aside.

3. Blend the almonds, walnuts, and sunflower seeds together in a food processor or a blender until it resembles coarse breadcrumbs. Add in the cooked broccoli and cauliflower. Blend until all the ingredients are finely chopped and well mixed. Add in the 1/2 cup mashed squash, cumin, salt, and pepper. Blend until well incorporated. If the mix is too thick to mix, transfer the ingredients into a bowl and mix hand.

4. Divide the mix into four equal portions and form into patties. In a large skillet, heat oil over medium-high heat. Cook the patties about 2 minutes each side, until heated through and browned. Enjoy with your favorite Paleo-friendly burger bun with avocado, lettuce, and tomato.

Stir-Fried Kale with Bacon

This yummy one-pan recipe is-fast and super easy to make. The bacon and vinegar perfectly balance the taste of the wilted bitter kale. You will definitely love this delicious shortcut to enjoy your greens.

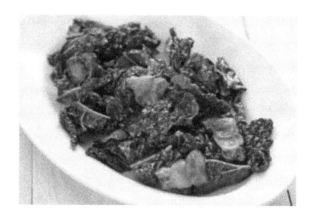

Prep Time: 10 minutes
Cook Time: 20 minutes

Serving Size: 170 g
Makes: 2
Calories: 472
Total Fat: 37.4 g
Saturated Fat: 10.6 g
Trans Fat: 0 g
Protein: 23.7 g
Net Carbs: 8.7 g
Total Carbs: 10 g
Dietary Fibre: 1.3 g
Sugars: 0 g
Cholesterol: 62 mg

Sodium: 1427 mg
Potassium: 756 mg
Vitamin A: 26%
Vitamin C: 181%
Calcium: 12%
Iron: 12%

Ingredients

- 4 ounces (about 1/2 cup) bacon, cut into 1/4-inch strips
- 1 bunch (about 6 ounces) kale, leaves removed, thinly chopped
- 2 tablespoons vegetable oil
- A squeeze of lemon
- Black pepper, freshly ground
- Kosher salt

Directions

1. In a large cast iron skillet, sauté the bacon bits with the oil over medium heat until they are crisp.

2. Add in the kale. Season with dash of salt and pepper. Stir the bacon and the kale for a few minutes. Add a splash of vinegar. Serve with a squeeze of lemon.

Chicken Salad Basilica

This recipe is another great way to enjoy your cauliflower rice. Who said you can't enjoy cauliflower for more than rice substitute? This new low carb meal is versatile and you can will find more to incorporate cauliflower rice in your keto life.

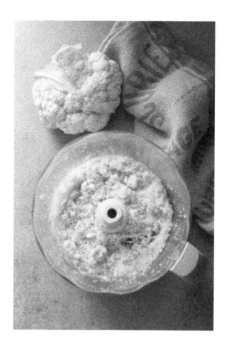

Prep Time: 10 minutes
Cook Time: 20 minutes

Serving Size: 180 g
Makes: 2
Calories: 414
Total Fat: 37.1 g
Saturated Fat: 6.6 g
Trans Fat: 0 g
Protein: 17.1 g

Net Carbs: 1.4 g
Total Carbs: 7 g
Dietary Fibre: 2.2 g
Sugars: 2.1 g
Cholesterol: 37 mg
Sodium: 390 mg
Potassium: 293 mg
Vitamin A: 9%
Vitamin C: 32%
Calcium: 17%
Iron: 10%

Ingredients

- 1/2 cup chicken, cooked, diced
- 2 tablespoons sun-dried tomatoes, packed in olive oil, chopped
- 2 tablespoons red wine vinegar
- 2 tablespoons pine nuts
- 2 tablespoons Parmesan cheese, shredded
- 1/4 head cauliflower, the bottom stems trimmed, cut into chunks
- 1/4 cup red onion, diced
- 1/4 cup olives, chopped (half green and half black)
- 1/4 cup olive oil, extra-virgin
- 1/4 cup fresh basil, minced
- 1 garlic clove, crushed
- Black pepper, ground
- Salt
- Water

Directions

1. Put the garlic into a small bowl. Pour in the olive oil. Allow to sit while you assemble the salad Put the cauliflower into the food processor and shred until rice grain size. Transfer into a microwavable bowl with a cover. Add a couple of teaspoons of water.

2. Cover the bowl; microwave for 4–5 minutes on high. When the microwave beeps, immediately remove the cover to stop further cooking. Drain the excess water and transfer into a large mixing bowl. Allow to cool for a couple of minutes.

3. In a small skillet over low heat, stir in the pine nuts until they are lightly golden. Add the basil, onion, olives, tomatoes, chicken, and pine nuts into the cauliflower bowl. Pour the garlic-infused olive oil over. Stir everything to mix.

4. Add in the vinegar. Stir everything again; season with salt and pepper to taste. Divide the salad between 2 plates. Top each serve with the Parmesan cheese.

Spinach with Bacon, Mushrooms, and Shallots

Well, you have probably noticed by now how we love to add bacon to our greens. And you probably also discovered that everything is better with bacon. It certainly packs a flavorful punch to sautéed spinach.

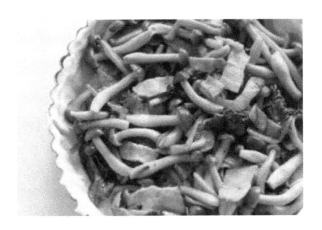

Prep Time: 10 minutes
Cook Time: 30 minutes

Serving Size: 450 g
Makes: 2
Calories: 415
Total Fat: 33.4 g
Saturated Fat: 12.6 g
Trans Fat: 0 g
Protein: 14.5 g
Net Carbs: 6.6 g
Total Carbs: 17.1 g
Dietary Fibre: 6 g
Sugars: 3.9 g

Cholesterol: 38 mg
Sodium: 454 mg
Potassium: 2119 mg
Vitamin A: 428%
Vitamin C: 108%
Calcium: 26%
Iron: 40%

Ingredients

- 12 ounces cremini mushrooms, sliced
- 1 pound baby spinach, organic
- 3 slices uncured bacon, baked and crumbled
- 2 teaspoons vinegar
- 2 large shallots, thinly sliced
- 4 tablespoons bacon grease, reserved from cooked bacon
- Black pepper, freshly ground
- Kosher salt

Directions

1. In a cast iron, over medium heat, heat the bacon grease. When hot, sauté the shallots with a dash of salt and pepper until they are soft and translucent.

2. Add in the mushrooms. Cook until they are browned and the mushroom liquid is evaporated. In batches, toss in the spinach, adding more as they wilt; season with vinegar, salt, and pepper. Plate the dish. Sprinkle with the bacon bits.

Big-O Burger

Warning: This burger is dangerously delicious. Your family and friends will be coming over to your house all the time for them. The bacon and the added mushrooms give the patties a powerful blast of flavors. Eat them wrapped in lettuce, or if you have time, roasted Portobello mushroom caps.

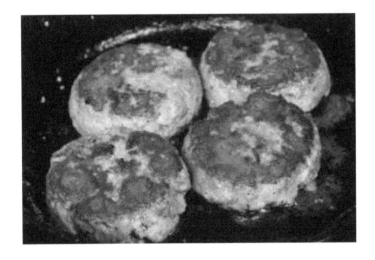

Prep Time: 30 minutes
Cook Time: 10 minutes

Serving Size: 221 g
Makes: 4
Calories: 470
Total Fat: 35.9 g
Saturated Fat: 9.2 g
Trans Fat: 0 g
Protein: 30.5 g
Net Carbs: 6.6 g
Total Carbs: 5.1 g

Dietary Fibre: 0.7 g
Sugars: 1.9 g
Cholesterol: 82 mg
Sodium: 1571 mg
Potassium: 897 mg
Vitamin A: 0%
Vitamin C: 0%
Calcium: 2%
Iron: 64%

Ingredients

- 4 ounces bacon, frozen, cross-cut into small pieces
- 1 pound ground beef
- 6 tablespoons vegetable oil, divided
- 1/2 pound cremini mushrooms, minced
- 1 1/2 teaspoons kosher salt
- Black pepper, freshly ground

Directions

1. In a cast-iron skillet over medium heat, heat 1 tablespoon of the ghee. Put the mushrooms. Sauté until the liquid has evaporated. Set aside and allow to cool to room temperature. Put the bacon in the food processor, pulse until ground meat in texture.

2. In a large mixing bowl, combine the mushrooms, bacon, and ground beef. Season with the salt and pepper. With your hands, gently combine the ingredients, making sure not to overwork the meat. Divide the mixture into 4

portions. Form each portion into balls and flatten into 3/4 –inch patties.

3. In a cast iron skillet over medium heat, heat the remaining 1 tablespoon oil. Cook the patties for about 3 minutes each side, turning once. When cooked, transfer to a wire rack to cool. Serve with your choice burger toppings, Portobello mushroom buns, or wrap them in lettuce leaves.

Cauliflower Fried Rice

Cauliflower rice is really a game changer. Gone are the days when you have to count calories every time you eat a dish with rice. This keto version is definitely a no-guilt Shortcut to Ketosis.

This lunch is all vegetables, but you won't know the difference since it definitely tastes like Chinese fried rice. Plus, if you have kids, they won't know they are eating cauliflower.

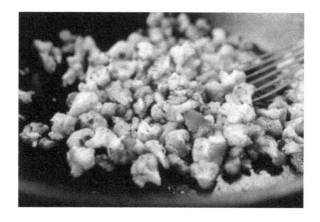

Prep Time: 15 minutes
Cook Time: 30 minutes

Serving Size: 176 g
Makes: 4
Calories: 217
Total Fat: 17.5 g
Saturated Fat: 9.4 g
Trans Fat: 0 g
Protein: 8.7 g
Net Carbs: 3.5 g

Total Carbs: 8.5 g
Dietary Fibre: 2.9 g
Sugars: 3.4 g
Cholesterol: 131 mg
Sodium: 711 mg
Potassium: 449 mg
Vitamin A: 15%
Vitamin C: 58%
Calcium: 5%
Iron: 13%

Ingredients

- 4 ounces mushrooms, sliced
- 3 slices bacon, uncured, cut into small dice
- 2 tablespoons cilantro leaves, chopped
- 2 tablespoons basil, chopped
- 2 scallions, thinly sliced
- 2 large eggs
- inch knob ginger, grated
- 1-2 tablespoons coconut aminos
- 1 tablespoon mint, chopped
- 1 small onion, minced
- 1 small head cauliflower, separated into florets
- 4 tablespoons ghee
- Black pepper, freshly ground
- Kosher salt

Optional

- Splash of fish sauce

- Splash of coconut vinegar

Directions

1. Put the cauliflower in a food processor. Process until the size of rice. In a large cast iron skillet, cook the bacon over medium heat until crispy. When cooked, transfer into a plate, leaving the grease into the skillet.

2. While the bacon is cooking, whisk the eggs in a small mixing bowl with some salt and pepper to taste. Pour on the skillet and cook until well done. When cooked, transfer to a plate and slice thinly. Set aside.

3. Increase the heat to medium high. Put in the onion. Season with a dash of salt and pepper. Cook until soft. Add in the mushrooms. Sprinkle with a dash of salt and pepper. Stir-fry until browned. Add in the ginger. Cook stirring for about 30 seconds.

4. Add in the cauliflower. Season with a dash of salt and pepper. Put the lid of the skillet. Lower the heat to low. Cook for about 5 minutes or until the cauliflower is tender but not mushy. Remove from the heat.

5. Add in the coconut aminos, herbs, and the eggs. If desired, add a splash of coconut vinegar and fish sauce. Add the bacon in. Toss everything together. Cream and top with the burger.

Tasty Tomato Soup

You'll definitely dive in head first to taste this creamy soup. It's so delicious you won't believe it's easy to make and low carb. The tomatoes and the aroma of the fresh basil come together beautifully fresh and vibrant. The tomatoes pack this soup with lycopene, which helps rid of free radicals that damage the cells of our body.

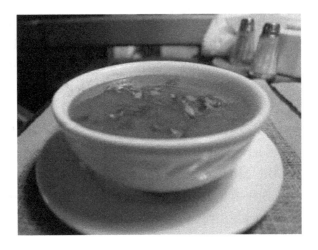

Prep Time: 15 minutes
Cook Time: 40 minutes

Serving Size: 519 g
Makes: 4
Calories: 319
Total Fat: 25.5 g
Saturated Fat: 7.5 g
Trans Fat: 0 g
Protein: 7 g
Net Carbs: 13.6 g
Total Carbs: 18.4 g

Dietary Fibre: 4.8 g
Sugars: 10.6 g
Cholesterol: 0 mg
Sodium: 613 mg
Potassium: 940 mg
Vitamin A: 143%
Vitamin C: 63%
Calcium: 9%
Iron: 9%

Ingredients

- 5 large tomatoes; chop roughly
- 3 garlic cloves; mince
- 3 cups vegetable or chicken broth
- 6 tablespoon vegetable oil
- 2 carrots; chop roughly
- 1 tablespoon tomato paste
- 1 large white onion; chop roughly
- ¼ cup fresh basil, chopped
- ¼ cup coconut milk

To taste

- Sea salt
- Freshly ground black pepper

Directions

1. In a large saucepan, heat cooking oil over medium heat. Add the onion in and the carrot. Cook for about 10

minutes or until soft. Add in the garlic. Cook for about 1-2 minutes more.

2. Add in the tomatoes, the tomato paste, the basil, and the chicken broth. Season with salt and pepper. Stir to combine ingredients.

3. Bring to boil. Adjust heat to low, simmer uncovered for about 30 minutes. Pour in the coconut milk. Blend the soup directly in the pan using immersion blender or blend using food processor until smooth.

Dinner Recipes

Steak with Mushroom Port Sauce

This go- to meal is easy to make and delicious. Just grab some piece of beef, cook it on a skillet, make the sauce in the same skillet, and you have a fancy dinner in almost no time at all. You also get to have fun flambéing the mushrooms.

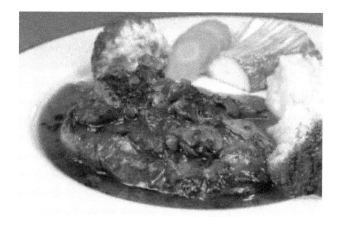

Prep Time: 10 minutes
Cook Time: 5-15 minutes

Serving Size: 688 g
Serves: 2
Calories: 1129
Total Fat: 39.3 g
Saturated Fat: 18 g
Trans Fat: 0 g
Protein: 4.5 g
Net Carbs: 5.6 g
Total Carbs: 7 g

Dietary Fibre: 1.4 g
Sugars: 2.9 g
Cholesterol: 462 mg
Sodium: 267 mg
Potassium: 2045 mg
Vitamin A: 12%
Vitamin C: 7%
Calcium: 4%
Iron: 107%

Ingredients

- 2 lb rib-eye steak
- 10 ounce. mushrooms
- 1 tablespoon of grass-fed butter
- Salt and pepper to taste
- 4 ounce. port wine
- 2 ounce. heavy cream

Directions

1. Preheat oven to 450F. Salt and pepper both sides of the steaks. Use a cast iron skillet and place on stove on high. Melt butter in skillet.

2. Cook steak for 2 minutes per side, and then move to the oven. Cook steak in the oven until internal temperature reaches desired level of doneness (135 for medium rare). When steaks are done, set aside and cover with tin foil.

3. Next, add some port wine to the pan and scrape off the burnt bits off the bottom. Add mushrooms and cream to

the skillet, then use a match to light wine on fire (optional). This will thicken the sauce, then pour over the steak and enjoy.

I hope you have learned something from this book so far and would greatly appreciate it if you could leave an honest review on Amazon.com

Pistachio-Crusted Salmon

Did you know that you can prepare a seriously sophisticated dinner within 20 minutes with just 6 ingredients? This recipe doesn't need fancy techniques or fussy ingredients to make it a crowd-pleasing meal.

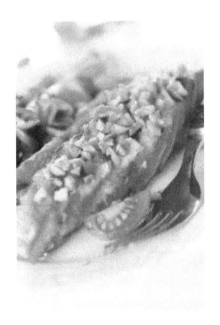

Prep Time: 5minutes
Cook Time: 15 minutes

Serving Size: 329 g
Serves: 2
Calories: 714
Total Fat: 56.9 g
Saturated Fat: 9.5 g
Trans Fat: 0 g
Protein: 49.2 g
Net Carbs: 13.6 g

Total Carbs: 7 g
Dietary Fibre: 3.2 g
Sugars: 1.5 g
Cholesterol: 100 mg
Sodium: 791 mg
Potassium: 1108 mg
Vitamin A: 6%
Vitamin C: 3%
Calcium: 13%
Iron: 16%

Ingredients

- pound wild king salmon fillet, skin on, pin bones removed
- 2 tablespoon scallions or chives, chopped
- 1/2 cup pistachios, shelled, salted, dry roasted, crushed
- 6 tablespoons Dijon mustard
- 5 tablespoons vegetable oil
- Black pepper, freshly ground
- Kosher salt

Directions

1. Preheat the 400F. Line a baking tray with parchment paper. With a paper towel, pat the fish dry. Divide the fillet into 2 uniform pieces. Season the skin with salt and pepper. With the skin-side down, lay it down on the prepared baking tray.

2. In a small mixing bowl, combine the mustard, vegetable oil, and the chives. Spread 1/2 of the mixture evenly on

each piece of fish. Sprinkle the crushed nuts on top of the mustard, patting them down gently and making sure they stick.

3. Place the tray in the oven. Bake for about 10-15 minutes or until the salmon is cooked through to your desired doneness. Remove the salmon from the oven. Allow to rest for a couple of minutes. Meanwhile, reheat some leftover vegetables and dice some cherry tomatoes.

Zoodles with Lamb Meatballs

Zucchini noodles or zoodles are what's in right now. You'll be surprised at how they make an excellent substitute for regular noodles. Use the julienne blade o fa trusty mandoline or a spiralizer. Top your zoodle with this scrumptious meatball recipe and enjoy a high taste, low-carb dinner.

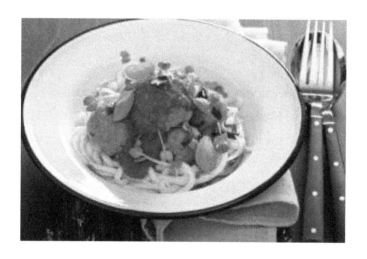

Prep Time: 10 minutes
Cook Time: 20 minutes

Serving Size: 306 g
Serves: 4
Calories: 676
Total Fat: 52.8 g
Saturated Fat: 12 g
Trans Fat: 0 g
Protein: 35 g
Net Carbs: 12.2 g
Total Carbs: 15.4 g
Dietary Fibre: 3.2 g

Sugars: 8.6 g
Cholesterol: 156 mg
Sodium: 444 mg
Potassium: 833 mg
Vitamin A: 14%
Vitamin C: 20%
Calcium: 6%
Iron: 23%

Ingredients

- 1/2 lb. (1 ounce.) zoodles (zucchini noodles)
- 12 ounce. Pasta sauce
- 1 lb. Ground lamb
- 2 shallots
- 1 egg yolk
- 1 teaspoon cinnamon
- 1 teaspoon cumin
- 12 tablespoons vegetable oil
- Cayenne pepper to taste
- Salt and pepper to taste
- Red pepper flakes to taste

Directions

1. Preheat oven to 450 degrees. Using a mandolin at the julienne setting, slice the zucchini. You only want the outer parts. Mix the rest of the ingredients together except for the pasta sauce and the olive oil and form 16 meatballs.

2. Cook the meatballs for 12 minutes in the oven. Stir the pasta sauce and oil together. Add the pasta sauce and zoodles into a saucepan and cook for an additional 3–4 minutes.

Turkey Curry in a Hurry

This quick to make dinner meal is a great use for any leftover turkey. This recipe transforms boring leftover meat into an exciting spicy dinner served over cauliflower rice or shirataki noodles.

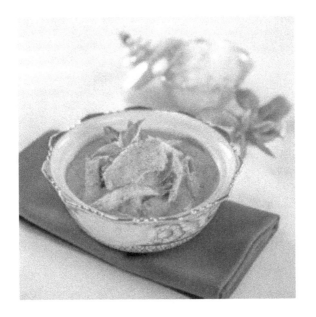

Prep Time: 10 minutes
Cook Time: 20 minutes

Serving Size: 222 g
Serves: 6
Calories: 476
Total Fat: 37.6 g
Saturated Fat: 19.5 g
Trans Fat: 0 g
Protein: 29.9 g
Net Carbs: 4.3 g

Total Carbs: 6.5 g
Dietary Fibre: 2.2 g
Sugars: 2.9 g
Cholesterol: 71 mg
Sodium: 201 mg
Potassium: 535 mg
Vitamin A: 3%
Vitamin C: 6%
Calcium: 2%
Iron: 61%

Ingredients

- 4 cups turkey, cooked, diced
- 3/4 cup chicken broth, or turkey broth if you have it
- 7 tablespoons vegetable oil (or coconut oil)
- 2 teaspoons garam masala
- 2 garlic cloves, crushed
- 1/2 medium onion, chopped
- 1 teaspoon ground turmeric
- 1 teaspoon ground cinnamon
- 1 teaspoon cayenne pepper
- 1 tablespoon fresh ginger, grated
- 1 3/4 cups (about 410 ml) coconut milk
- Salt

Directions

1. In a big, heavy skillet over medium-low heat, add the oil. Add in the garam masala, turmeric, and cinnamon. Stir

for 1 minute or so. Add in the onions. Sauté until translucent.

2. Add the coconut milk, the chicken broth, ginger, garlic, and cayenne. Stir until the sauce becomes creamy. Stir in the turkey. Adjust the burner to low. Simmer for about 15 minutes. Season with salt to taste. Serve over cauliflower rice or shirataki noodles.

Salmon with Mango-Avocado Salsa

If you love tropical fruits, you'll crave this recipe! The mango-avocado salsa topped on pan-seared salmon gives this dish a refreshing tangy taste.

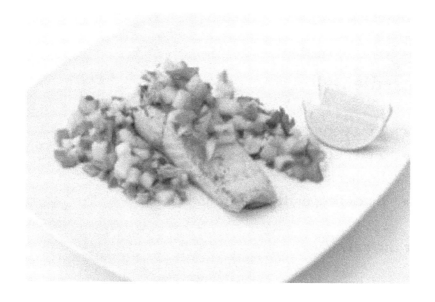

Prep Time: 20 minutes
Cook Time: 10 minutes

Serving Size: 250 g
Serves: 5
Calories: 487
Total Fat: 38.9 g
Saturated Fat: 8.4 g
Trans Fat: 0 g
Protein: 27.3 g
Net Carbs: 8 g
Total Carbs: 11 g
Dietary Fibre: 3 g

Sugars: 6.8 g
Cholesterol: 73 mg
Sodium: 95 mg
Potassium: 757 mg
Vitamin A: 14%
Vitamin C: 28%
Calcium: 6%
Iron: 6%

Ingredients

- 1 1/2 pounds fresh wild king salmon filet
- 2 tablespoons ghee
- Kosher salt
- Black pepper, freshly ground

For the salsa

- 7 tablespoons olive oil, extra virgin
- 2 cups (about 2 mangos) ripe mango, diced
- 1/4 teaspoon red pepper flakes
- 1/4 cup fresh cilantro, minced
- 1/2 cup red onion, finely diced
- 1 cup (1 medium avocado) Hass avocado, diced
- 1 lime, juiced
- Black pepper, freshly ground

Directions

For the salmon

1. Cut the salmon into 5 serving pieces. Pat the fish with a paper towel until very dry. Season all the sides with salt and pepper. In a cast iron skillet over medium-high heat, heat the ghee until simmering.

2. With the skin side down, put in the salmon fillets. Turn down the heat to medium-low. Gently press each fillet down with a flexible spatula to prevent them from curling up and the skin to crisp evenly.

3. Cook for about 6 minutes or until the skin easily comes off the surface of the skillet or the meat thermometer is between 120F–130F. Quickly sear the meat sides for about 30 seconds each. Place on the plate with the crispy skin on top. Top each serve with salsa.

For the salsa

1. Put the diced mango in a bowl. Add in the rest of the ingredients. Stir to combine.

2. Adjust the seasoning according to taste; top over the salmon fillets.

Shrimp-Stuffed Mushrooms

Whenever I serve this dish, there are never any leftovers. They are incredibly delicious bites. The seafood stuffing takes the meaty, rich flavor and texture of the mushrooms to another level of deliciousness!

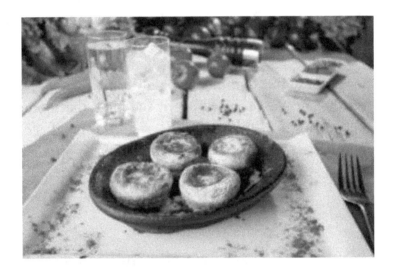

Prep Time: 20 minutes
Cook Time: 20 minutes

Serving Size: 356 g
Serves: 3 (8 pieces each)
Calories: 493
Total Fat: 39 g
Saturated Fat: 11.6g
Trans Fat: 0 g
Protein: 24.8 g
Net Carbs: 9.7 g
Total Carbs: 11.4 g
Dietary Fibre: 1.7 g

Sugars: 4.2 g
Cholesterol: 186 mg
Sodium: 502 mg
Potassium: 1209 mg
Vitamin A: 14%
Vitamin C: 5%
Calcium: 12%
Iron: 8%

Ingredients

- 8 ounces shrimp, frozen or fresh, thawed if frozen
- 24 ounces (about 24 pieces medium-sized) cremini mushrooms
- 2 bacon slices (about 1/3 cup), diced
- 2 tablespoons ghee
- 1/4 cup scallions (about 2 scallions), roughly chopped
- 1/4 cup cilantro, packed
- 1 teaspoon fish sauce
- 1 tablespoon jalapeño pepper, diced small
- 6 tablespoons vegetable oil
- Black pepper, freshly ground
- Kosher salt

Directions

1. Preheat the oven to 450F. Clean and remove the stems of the mushrooms. With the gill-side down, put the mushrooms into a foil-lined baking sheet. Brush them with the melted ghee. Roast for about 12 minutes.

2. Flip the mushrooms over and roast for about 5–10 minutes more or until the mushroom liquid has evaporated. While the mushrooms are roasting, de-vein and remove the tails of the shrimp. Chop them into medium-sized pieces.

3. In the work bowl of a food processor, toss the shrimp with the bacon, cilantro, scallions, jalapeño pepper, vegetable oil, and fish sauce; season with the salt and pepper. Process the ingredients until it turns into a coarsely chopped texture with a pasty, sticky chunky mixture.

4. With a small dish or spoon, scoop out the filling and fill each mushroom with the paste. Return the mushroom into the oven; cook for about 8-10 minutes or until the mixture is set. Serve topped with Sriracha, if desired.

Bacon and Cheddar Fritters

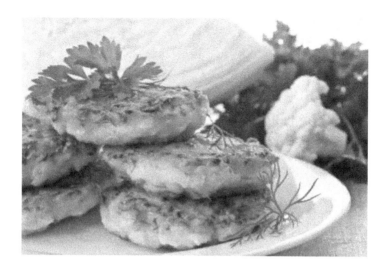

Preparation time: 10 minutes
Cooking time: 15 minutes

Serves: 6
Total Carbohydrates: 5g
Dietary Fiber: 2g
Net Cabs: 3g
Protein: 13g
Total Fat: 16g
Calories: 223

Ingredients

- ⅔ cup cooked and crumbled bacon
- 1 ½ cups grated cheddar cheese
- 1 medium head cauliflower
- 3 large eggs
- 3 tablespoons coconut flour

- 2 cloves garlic, minced
- Sea salt and pepper to taste
- Coconut oil for the pan

Directions

1. Chop the cauliflower into ½-inch pieces and steam for about 10–15 minutes, until soft. Drain well and mash with a fork or potato masher, pressing to release as much liquid as possible. Transfer the cauliflower to a large bowl. Add the eggs, cheese, bacon, garlic, and coconut flour. Season with salt and pepper and mix well.

2. Heat a large skillet over medium heat and add about a tablespoon of coconut oil. Form the cauliflower mixture into flat patties, using about 2–3 tablespoons per patty.

3. Once the pan is hot, add a few of the patties and cook for 3–5 minutes, until browned on the bottom. Flip carefully and cook another 3–5 minutes. Remove to a paper towel-lined plate and repeat with the remaining patties. Serve hot.

***Trivia:** One serving of cauliflower contains 77% of your daily recommended amount of vitamin C. It's also a good source of fiber, potassium, and protein, believe it or not!*

Chicken and Mushroom Cream Crepes

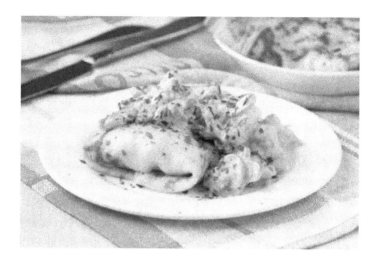

Preparation time: 10 minutes
Cooking time: 25 minutes

Serves: 4
Total Carbohydrates: 5g
Dietary Fiber: 1g
Net Carbs: 4g
Protein: 29g
Total Fat: 43g
Calories: 518

Ingredients

- 1 boneless, skinless chicken breast, cut into ½-inch pieces
- 1 cup sliced mushrooms
- 2 cups heavy cream
- 4 large eggs

- 1 yellow onion, thinly sliced
- 4 slices bacon, cooked and chopped
- Sea salt and pepper to taste
- Olive oil for the pan
- Optional garnish: chopped parsley and/or chives

Directions

1. Whisk the eggs together with about a tablespoon of heavy cream and season with salt and pepper. Heat a small pan over medium heat and add a bit of olive oil to it. Pour approximately ½ cup of the egg mixture to the pan and swirl to evenly coat the pan.

2. Once the eggs have set, flip and cook for about 1 minute. Transfer to a paper towel and repeat 3 times with the remaining egg mixture.

3. In a large pan, sauté the chicken, onions, and mushrooms together until the chicken is cooked through. Season with salt and pepper. Stir in the bacon and the heavy cream. Cook about 3–4 minutes, until slightly thickened. Divide most the chicken mixture between the 4 egg crepes, fold, and top with the remaining cream. Serve and enjoy!

Trivia: For thousands of years, mushrooms have been celebrated as a powerful source for nutrients. They are a good source of B vitamins, which play an important role in the nervous system. They also contain high amounts of selenium, a mineral that is important to the immune system.

Italian Breakfast

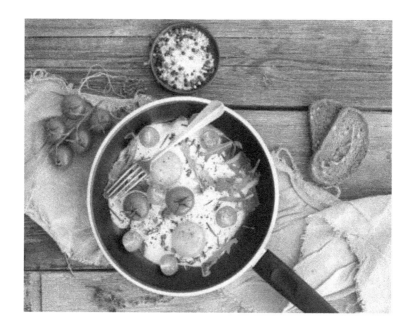

Preparation time: 5 minutes
Cooking time: 12 minutes

Serves: 4
Total Carbohydrates: 5g
Dietary Fiber: 3g
Net Carbs: 2g
Protein: 11g
Total Fat: 19g
Calories: 228

Ingredients

- 4 large eggs
- 4 slices prosciutto ham

- 12 cherry tomatoes, halved
- 2 cloves garlic, minced
- 1 cup rocket lettuce
- 4 tablespoons of butter
- Sea salt and black pepper to taste

Directions

1. Heat 2 tablespoons of butter in a large skillet on a medium-high heat. Crack and fry the eggs, preferably sunny side up, until the edges are golden (usually around 3–4 minutes). Remove from the pan and set aside for the moment.

2. Add the remaining butter, then add the garlic to the skillet and sauté until it begins to turn golden brown. Add the cherry tomatoes and sauté for 3–4 minutes. Layer the prosciutto and rocket lettuce on top of the tomatoes. Top with the precooked eggs.

3. Cover and allow everything to warm through for 2–3 minutes. Season with additional salt and pepper, if desired, and serve immediately.

Baked Eggs with Hollandaise

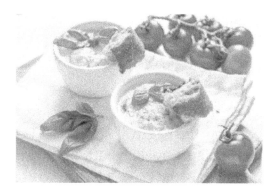

Preparation time: 10 minutes
Cooking time: 20 minutes

Serves: 4
Total Carbohydrates: 2g
Dietary Fiber: 1g
Net Carbs: 1g
Protein: 24g
Total Fat: 34g
Calories: 411

Ingredients

- 4 strips of bacon, chopped
- 2 cups baby spinach or kale
- 8 large eggs
- Optional garnish: fresh basil

Hollandaise Sauce

- 2 egg yolks

- ¼ cup butter, melted
- 1 tablespoon lemon juice
- ¼ teaspoon salt

Directions

1. To prepare the hollandaise sauce: In a high-speed blender, blend the egg yolks with the lemon juice and salt. Slowly pour the melted butter into the blender while it's running. Blend for about 30 seconds, until thickened. Pour into a small bowl set over a sauce pan of simmering water to keep warm until ready to use.

2. For the baked eggs: Preheat oven to 400°F. Position the rack in the top third of the oven. Heat a large skillet over medium heat. Cook the bacon until crisp. Add the greens and sauté until wilted. Divide the mixture evenly between 4 large ramekins or gratin dishes.

3. Gently crack 2 eggs onto the filling of each ramekin. Place on a baking sheet and into the oven for 10–12 minutes, until the white is set, but the yolk is still runny.

4. Drizzle with hollandaise sauce, garnish with fresh basil, if desired, and serve immediately. I cannot help but to serve this dish with a couple of 'soldiers'. The yolks are great for dipping a couple of sticks of low-carb bread into.

Trivia: Hollandaise sauce is a simple emulsion of egg yolk and butter that is widely used in French cooking. It adds a creamy richness to the eggs in this recipe. If you'd like to spice it up a bit, try adding a pinch of cayenne pepper to it before blending.

Slow Cooker Sausage Stuffed Peppers

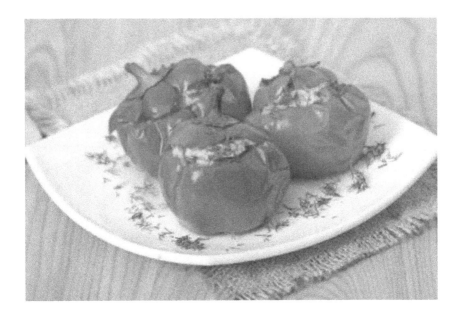

Preparation time: 10 minutes
Cooking time: 6 hours

Serves: 4
Total Carbohydrates: 18g
Dietary Fiber: 6g
Net Carbs: 12g
Protein: 27g
Total Fat: 33g
Calories: 485

Ingredients:

- 1 pound Italian sausage
- 4 bell peppers
- ½ head of cauliflower

- 1 (8 ounce) can tomato paste
- 1 small yellow onion, diced
- 3 garlic cloves, minced
- 2 teaspoons oregano
- Sea salt and pepper to taste

Directions:

1. Cut the tops off of the bell peppers and discard the seeds. Save the tops. Grate the cauliflower into "rice" with a cheese grater or food processor and transfer to a large mixing bowl. Add the minced garlic, oregano, and onion. Mix well to combine.

2. Add the sausage and tomato paste to the cauliflower mixture and mix well with your hands. Season with salt and pepper. Evenly divide the sausage mixture between the peppers. Cover each pepper with their tops and gently place into your slow cooker. Cook on low for 6 hours. Serve and enjoy!

Trivia: Bell peppers have quite a bit going for them. They're low in calories, high in fiber, and an excellent source of vitamins A and C.

Blueberry Coffee Cake

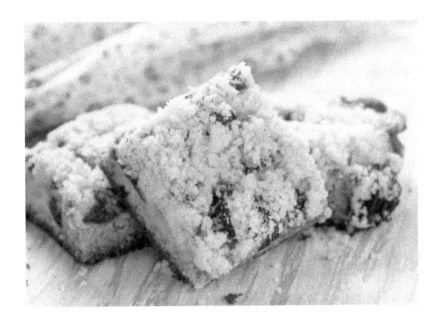

Preparation time: 15 minutes
Cooking time: 30 minutes

Serves: 6
Total Carbohydrates: 6g
Dietary Fiber: 2g
Net Carbs: 4g
Protein: 6g
Total Fat: 26g
Calories: 270

Ingredients

- 1 cup fresh or frozen blueberries (or other berry of choice)
- 4 large eggs, separated

- ½ cup coconut flour
- ¼ cup coconut oil
- ¼ cup sugar substitute
- 2 teaspoons vanilla extract
- ¼ teaspoon baking soda
- 1 teaspoon cream of tartar

Topping

- ¼ cup coconut sugar
- ¼ cup coconut oil
- 2 tablespoons coconut flour
- ½ teaspoon cinnamon

Directions

1. Preheat oven to 350°F. Prepare an 8x8 baking pan with non-stick spray. In a large bowl, combine the egg whites and cream of tartar. Whisk until stiff peaks form.

2. In another bowl, cream together the sugar substitute and coconut oil. Mix in the egg yolks. Slowly stir in the coconut flour, vanilla, and baking soda. Mix until just combined. Gently fold the egg whites into the batter. Pour into the prepared pan. Evenly scatter the blueberries on top.

3. In a small bowl, mix the ingredients for the topping. Spread the mixture over the batter. Bake for 30 minutes, or until a toothpick inserted comes out clean.

Allow to cool to room temperature before cutting into squares.

Trivia: *Coconut flour is a versatile kitchen staple that's popular in the keto community. It's high in fiber and a great source of heart-healthy fats.*

Garam Masala Meatballs with Apple Chutney

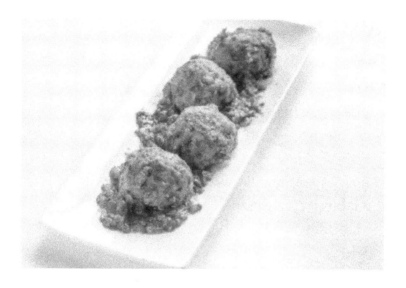

Preparation time: 15 minutes
Cooking time: 30 minutes

Serves: 4
Total Carbohydrates: 18g
Dietary Fiber: 3g
Net Carbs: 15g
Protein: 16g
Total Fat: 12g
Calories: 249

Ingredients

For the Meatballs

- ½ pound lean ground pork

- 1 teaspoon onion powder
- 1 teaspoon salt
- 1 teaspoon garam masala

For the Apple Chutney

- 2 medium tart apples (such as Granny Smith)
- ¼ cup raisins
- 2 tablespoons butter
- ½ teaspoon garam masala
- 1 tablespoon maple syrup
- 2 tablespoons water
- 1 tablespoon apple cider vinegar

Directions

1. Preheat oven to 400°F. Line a baking sheet with parchment paper. In a large bowl, combine all of the meatball ingredients. Mix well with hands. Portion into small balls and bake for about 15–20 minutes, until cooked through.

2. To prepare the chutney: Combine all of the ingredients into a medium saucepan over medium heat. Bring to a simmer, cover, and allow to cook for 6–8 minutes, stirring occasionally. Mash the chutney with a potato masher or fork until few chunks remain. Top the meatballs with the chutney and enjoy.

Trivia: *Garam masala is an aromatic blend of ground spices common in Indian cuisine. It can be found in the international aisle of most grocery stores.*

Egg-Stuffed Breakfast Meatloaf

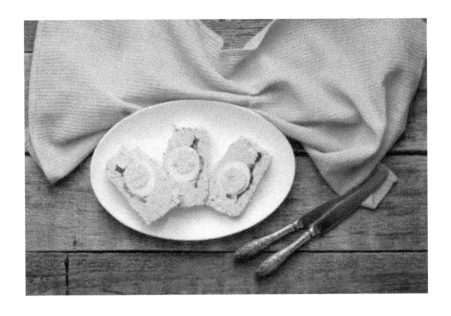

Preparation time: 15 minutes
Cooking time: 35 minutes

Serves: 6
Total Carbohydrates: 0g
Dietary Fiber: 2g
Net Carbs: 0g
Protein: 33g
Total Fat: 7g
Calories: 204g

Ingredients

- 4 hardboiled eggs, peeled
- 1 cup baby spinach or kale
- 1 ½ pounds ground pork

- 1 teaspoon smoked paprika
- 1 teaspoon fennel seeds
- ½ teaspoon salt
- ½ teaspoon pepper
- ½ teaspoon sage
- ¼ teaspoon cayenne pepper

Directions

1. Preheat oven to 400°F. Prepare a 9x5 inch loaf pan with non-stick spray. In a large mixing bowl, combine the ground pork with the spices and mix well with hands. Place a thin layer of pork in the bottom of the prepared pan.

2. Line the baby spinach down the center of the pan and top with the hard-boiled eggs. Place the remaining pork on top and press gently. Bake for 35 minutes, or until golden brown. Allow to cool for 5–10 minutes. Slice and serve.

Trivia: Meatloaf doesn't have to be just for dinner. This savory breakfast meatloaf is a unique spin on eggs and sausage. Individual slices can be wrapped tightly in plastic wrap and stored in the freezer for several weeks.

Don't forget to share your thoughts on this book by leaving a review on Amazon.com. It takes just a few seconds.

Sweet Potato-Crusted Veggie Frittata

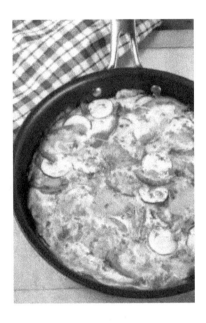

Preparation time: 15 minutes
Cooking time: 60 minutes

Serves: 6
Total Carbohydrates: 14g
Dietary Fiber: 3g
Net Carbs: 11g
Protein: 9g
Total Fat: 12g
Calories: 212

Ingredients

- 2 sweet potatoes, peeled and very thinly sliced
- 1 medium zucchini, sliced
- 1 bell pepper, sliced

- 2 cups baby spinach
- 3 bacon slices, cooked and crumbled (reserve about 1 tablespoon of the fat)
- 1 small onion, sliced
- 5 eggs, beaten
- 2 tablespoons olive oil
- 2 cloves garlic, minced
- Sea salt and pepper to taste

Directions

1. Preheat oven to 400°F. Toss the sweet potato slices with olive oil and season with salt and pepper. Arrange the slices in a 9" pie dish to form a crust for the quiche. Bake for 15–20 minutes.

2. While the crust bakes, add the reserved bacon fat to a large skillet over medium heat. Sauté the garlic, zucchini, bell pepper and onion until translucent. Add the spinach and cook until wilted. Remove from heat. Once the sweet potatoes are done, lower the heat to 375°F.

3. Layer the spinach mixture into the crust, top with the beaten eggs and crumbled bacon. Season with salt and pepper and bake for 30–35 minutes, until the eggs are set. Serve warm.

Trivia: Eating deep orange-colored fruits and vegetables, such as sweet potatoes, is associated with lower risk of coronary heart disease. A good reason to include them in your regular diet!

Cheddar, Chorizo & Green Chile Breakfast Bake

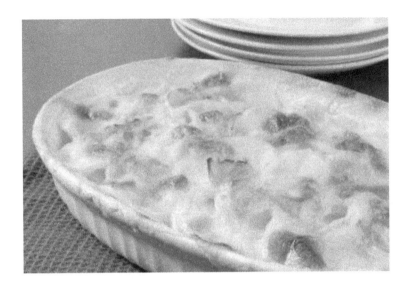

Preparation time: 15 minutes
Cooking time: 45 minutes

Serves: 6
Total Carbohydrates: 22g
Dietary Fiber: 12g
Net Carbs: 10g
Protein: 23g
Total Fat: 27g
Calories: 430

Ingredients

- 1 pound chorizo sausage
- 1 (8 ounce) can green chilies
- 1 cup shredded cheddar cheese

- 1 yellow onion, diced
- ½ head cauliflower
- 4 eggs, beaten
- ½ teaspoon garlic powder
- Sea salt and pepper to taste
- Optional garnish: sliced green onions

Directions

1. Preheat oven to 375°F. Grease a 9x13 glass baking dish with olive oil. In a skillet over medium heat, cook the chorizo and onion until golden brown. Add the chilies to the pan and mix well. Transfer to a large mixing bowl and allow to cool slightly.

2. Shred the cauliflower into "rice" using a food processor or cheese grater. Add to the bowl. Stir in the beaten eggs and half of the cheese. Season with salt, pepper, and garlic salt. Pour into the prepared dish. Top with the remaining cheese.

3. Bake for 45 minutes, until the eggs are set and cheese is golden brown. Let rest for 5 minutes. Top with green onions, if desired. Serve!

Trivia: *Chorizo is a pork sausage that is heavily seasoned with paprika and other spices. It can be found in most grocery stores, but regular breakfast sausage can be substituted, if it's not available in your area.*

Deviled Eggs

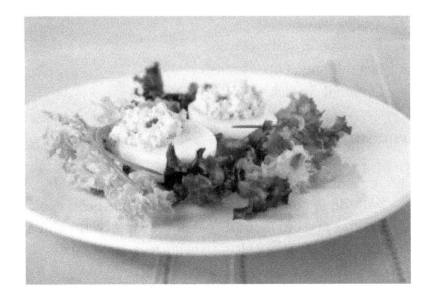

Preparation time: 15 minutes
Cooking time: 10 minutes

Serves: 4
Total Carbohydrates: 2g
Dietary Fiber: 0g
Net Carbs: 2g
Protein: 11g
Total Fat: 19g
Calories: 217

Ingredients

- 8 hardboiled eggs, peeled and sliced in half
- 1 tablespoon mayonnaise
- 1 teaspoon Dijon mustard

- 1 tablespoon heavy cream
- 1 tablespoon olive oil
- 1 clove garlic, minced
- 1 tablespoon green onion, minced
- 1 teaspoon lemon juice
- 2 tablespoons parsley, roughly chopped

Directions

1. Gently remove the yolks from the hard-boiled eggs and place in a medium bowl. Place the whites on a serving tray. Add the mayonnaise, mustard, heavy cream, olive oil, garlic, green onion, lemon juice, and parsley.

2. Mash everything together until a thick paste forms. Spoon the mixture back into the egg whites. Serve over a bed of salad greens.

Trivia: The concept of deviled eggs began in Ancient Rome although the name is an 18th century invention. The word "deviled" was used to describe highly seasoned fried or boiled dishes.

Soft Boiled Eggs with Avocado Salsa

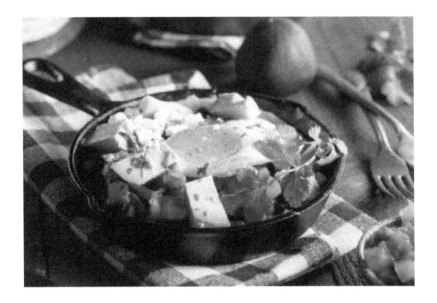

Preparation time: 15 minutes
Cooking time: 30 minutes

Serves: 4
Total Carbohydrates: 8g
Dietary Fiber: 4g
Net Carbs: 4g
Protein: 13g
Total Fat: 19g
Calories: 240

Ingredients

- 8 large eggs
- 1 avocado, diced
- 1 cup cherry tomatoes, quartered

- ¼ cup red onion, diced
- ½ cup cilantro, roughly chopped
- ½ a jalapeño, minced
- ¼ cup feta cheese
- ½ teaspoon sea salt
- Juice of 1 lime

Directions

1. To prepare the avocado salsa: Combine everything but the eggs in a medium bowl and mix well. Cover and refrigerate until ready to serve.

2. To soft boil the eggs: Fill a medium saucepan with water and bring to a boil. Reduce heat to a simmer and add the eggs to the pot. Cook 5 minutes for a runny yolk, or 7 minutes for a soft-set yolk. Remove from heat and run the eggs under cold water for about 1 minute, or until cool enough to peel. Gently peel the eggs and plate with a big scoop of the avocado salsa. Enjoy!

Trivia: *Soft boiled egg tip: Work in batches of 4 eggs at a time to avoid overcrowding the saucepan. Be sure to set a timer, they can go from soft boiled to hard boiled very quickly, if you're not paying attention.*

Keto Egg Casserole

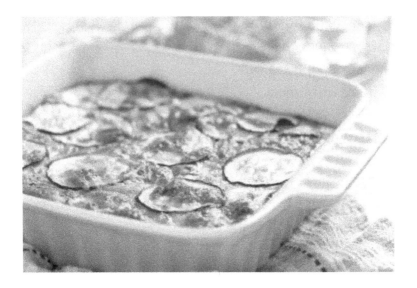

Preparation time: 10 minutes
Cooking time: 30 minutes

Serves: 6
Total Carbohydrates: 4g
Dietary Fiber: 1g
Net Carbs: 3g
Protein: 30g
Total Fat: 38g
Calories: 478

Ingredients

- 12 large eggs
- 1 pound breakfast sausage
- 1 zucchini, thinly sliced
- ½ red onion, diced

- ½ green pepper, diced
- 1 cup half & half
- ½ cup shredded cheddar cheese
- ¼ teaspoon thyme
- Sea salt and pepper to taste
- Optional garnish: chopped fresh basil leaves

Directions

1. Preheat oven to 350°F. Prepare an 8x8 baking dish with non-stick spray. In a large skillet over medium heat, brown the sausage. Once the sausage is cooked through, add the onions, peppers, and zucchini. Cook until tender. Remove from heat.

2. In a large bowl, whisk the eggs until frothy. Season with salt, pepper, and thyme. Add the vegetables to the eggs and pour into the prepared baking dish. Sprinkle evenly with the shredded cheese. Bake for 30 minutes, until the eggs are set. Garnish with chopped basil, if desired and serve.

Trivia: *This simple recipe can be adapted any way you like. Get creative and throw in whatever add-ins you'd like! Cheese, hot peppers, and black olives are all great choices. Add a fried egg on top for decoration when having friends over.*

Grilled Calamari & Roasted Peppers

This super easy and quick to flash-grilled calamari dinner meal is a great seafood dish. A tangy salad is perfect complement to this recipe.

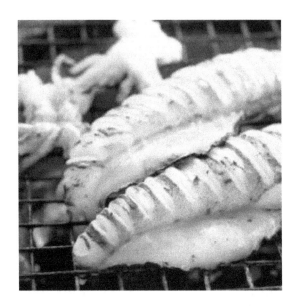

Prep Time: 30 minutes
Cook Time: 10 minutes

Serving Size: 257 g
Serves: 3
Calories: 451
Total Fat: 35.2 g
Saturated Fat: 8.9 g
Trans Fat: 0 g
Protein: 24.3 g
Net Carbs: 7.7 g
Total Carbs: 8.8 g
Dietary Fibre: 1.1 g

Sugars: 2 g
Cholesterol: 366 mg
Sodium: 146 mg
Potassium: 526 mg
Vitamin A: 36%
Vitamin C: 116%
Calcium: 6%
Iron: 9%

Ingredients

- 1 pound squid, cleaned, gutted
- 1 medium red bell pepper
- 2 small shallot, thinly sliced
- 2 tablespoon balsamic vinegar
- 2 tablespoon lemon juice, from 1 lemon
- 1/4 cup Italian parsley leaves
- 3 tablespoons bacon grease, melted or your fat of choice
- 4 tablespoons olive oil, extra virgin
- Black pepper, freshly ground
- Kosher salt

Directions

1. Place the bell pepper directly on your gas range. Turn on the heat and char it until the skin is black all over. Place the pepper in a bowl. Tightly cover with plastic wrap or foil. Let them steam for at least 15 minutes. Rub off the blackened skin. Remove the stems, seeds, and the ribs. Cut into strips. Set aside.

2. Gut the squids, rinse, and dry. Cut each one open so they would lie flat on the grill. Remove the skin if you desire. Toss the squid with the bacon grease; season with salt and pepper to taste.

3. In a small mixing bowl, combine the balsamic vinegar and the shallots. Allow to mellow out. Preheat the grill on high. When the grill is hot, cook the squid for about 20–30 seconds per side. The tentacles will take longer to cook. However, don't cook them for too long or they will turn to rubber.

4. When the squid is flash-grilled, slice it. Put in a bowl. Add the lemon juice and pour in the olive oil. Toss to coat evenly. Transfer to the balsamic-shallot mix.

5. Add the sliced pepper; season with salt and pepper. Mix everything well. Sprinkle with parsley. Taste and adjust lemon juice, salt, and pepper according to taste.

Orange Dijon Chicken

This chicken recipe makes a delicious bang using just a few ingredients. This home-made version of a restaurant-quality Dijon mustard marinade, makes for a zesty, sweet dish that's a hit for both kids and kids at heart.

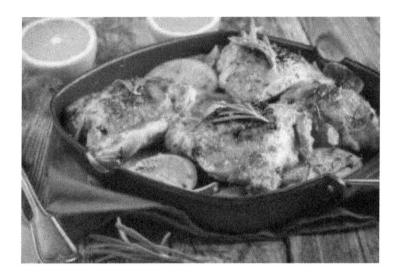

Prep Time: 5 minutes, plus marinating
Cook Time: 40 minutes

Serving Size: 414 g
Serves: 4
Calories: 629
Total Fat: 22.3 g
Saturated Fat: 5.5 g
Trans Fat: 0 g
Protein: 96.1 g
Net Carbs: 3.9 g
Total Carbs: 5.9 g
Dietary Fibre: 2 g

Sugars: 1.7 g
Cholesterol: 299 mg
Sodium: 1969 mg
Potassium: 816 mg
Vitamin A: 6%
Vitamin C: 26%
Calcium: 8%
Iron: 32%

Ingredients

- 3 pounds chicken thighs or drumsticks
- Italian parsley or chives, minced

For the marinade

- 1/4 cup orange juice, freshly squeezed
- 3/4 cup Dijon mustard
- 2 tablespoons avocado oil or extra virgin olive oil
- 6 garlic cloves, minced
- 2 teaspoons kosher salt

Directions

1. Preheat the oven to 425F or 400F for convection. Place the rack in the middle position. Line a rimmed baking sheet with aluminum foil. Place a stainless-steel wire rack on top.

2. In a large mixing bowl, combine all the marinade ingredients together, adjusting the amount of salt

according to taste. Mix well. Put the chicken into the marinade. Coat each piece well. If desired, marinade in the morning for dinner cooking. Don't marinade for more than a day.

3. Gently shake off excess marinade from the chicken. In a single layer, lay the drumsticks on the wire rack in the prepared baking sheet.

4. Roast for about 20 minutes. Flip the drumsticks over and rotate the tray 180 degrees. Continue roasting for 20 minutes more or until the meat is cooked to the internal temperature of 170F and the skin is browned. Serve with a sprinkle of parsley.

Discover Scientifically-Proven "Shortcuts" & "Hacks" to Lose Weight FASTER (With Very Little Effort)

For this month only, you can get Linda's best-selling & most popular book absolutely free – *Weight Loss Secrets You NEED to Know.*

Get Your FREE Copy Here:
TopFitnessAdvice.com/Bonus

Discover scientifically-proven tips to help you lose weight faster and easier than ever before. With this book, readers were able to improve their weight loss results and fitness levels. So, it's highly recommended that you get this book, especially while it's free!

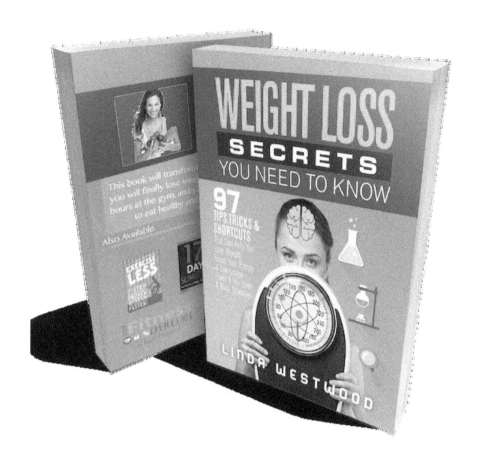

Get Your FREE Copy Here:
TopFitnessAdvice.com/Bonus

Conclusion

The Ketogenic Diet has existed in many variations over the years. In fact, it may have been the first diet humans have ever known. But the real question is: "Should I go for it?" Hopefully by this point the answer is no-brainer.

If you are still deciding if this diet is worth your time, the only question you should answer is "What do I have to lose?".

Making big changes in life is never easy. In fact, most people delay making changes until they need to.

If you're 25 and in shape, make a change so you're not 45 and overweight. If you're 45 and overweight, make a change so you're not 65 and diabetic. If you're 65 and diabetic, make a change so that you're still alive and healthy at 85! It's never too early, or too late to take control of your health.

The Ketogenic Diet is becoming more and more popular because it works. It is not a fad, and it is not a trend. Studies keep coming out that show the tremendous benefits of being on a low carb, high fat diet.

Even good ideas take time before mainstream culture recognizes its benefits. Take a car, for example. It is something today that is universally considered a pretty good idea. However, when it first came out people thought it was too smelly, too loud and too dangerous. A horse drawn carriage was considered to be a safer and more efficient mode of transportation!

There is a similar resistance to the idea of having a low carb diet. After all, fruits and vegetables are carbs! How can those be bad?

That is when scientific research come into play. It shows people on a Ketogenic Diet burn more fat per hour, and have lower blood pressure. It also shows people that are on it have an increase in good cholesterol and a decrease in bad cholesterol. With more and more research coming out there will be a point where the benefits of the diet are undeniable. So, it is better to start your journey on the road to greater health today.

There will of course be some challenges along the way. For example, most people look at you strange when you tell them you're on a low carb diet. You might as well be telling them that you entered a booger-eating contest and won first place! Because their reaction would be similar; half shock and half disgust.

If you want even more confusion, try telling a waiter that you're on a Ketogenic Diet and you can't have sugar in your salad dressing.
I found the easiest thing to tell people is that you're not eating carbs because you're trying to be healthy. In addition, tell the waiter you can't have any sugar because you're diabetic. Just make sure you know the difference between type 1 and type 2!

If you are just starting out just know that you may feel lethargic and weak the first week or two when you begin the diet. But don't be alarmed, just know that this is your body changing to a fat burning machine!

When you first start the Ketogenic Diet, it is best to avoid strenuous exercise for the first week or so. To help kick-start your weight loss go for a nice long walk. If you go to the gym often, keep the weights light and focus on easy cardio. Adding MCT Oil will also help you give you more energy during this period. But the most important thing to do is just be patient; and give your body time to adjust.

Remember to consume the majority of your calories from high quality fats and protein. Treat yourself every now and again with fresh fruit or a glass of wine. Make sure to limit your carbohydrate intake to about 20 to 60 grams per day.

Nevertheless, every person is different. Some people need to stay under 20 grams to enter ketosis. Others can go up to 80 grams and still get into ketosis. However, when starting out, keep carbs on the lower end.

If you are on the diet and become tempted to give up or have a really bad cheat meal, just focus on your priorities in life. Look at what you have achieved. Do you feel better? Are you losing weight? Remember that you are on the path to a better lifestyle.

When you have a setback, handle it immediately. If you eat or drink something that isn't on your diet, don't give up. The Ketogenic Diet is a lifestyle change. There will be occasions where you fall to temptation.

When you eat a certain amount of carbs you will come out of ketosis. Just be aware that it isn't the end of the world and it may just take you a couple of days to get back into the flow. It is easy to get caught off track, but once you are on the diet and notice all the positive effects it will be easy to get back.

You can help stay motivated by getting support from other Ketogenic Dieters. I recommend going on Facebook and typing in Ketogenic. There are many fantastic groups you can join with people that will inspire you daily. I would love to hear from you.

Just remember that the hardest part of this diet is the first few days. Once you get past that point things get much easier. So, think about your family, think about your friends, most importantly think about yourself, and never give up!

Final Words

I would like to thank you for purchasing my book and I hope I have been able to help you and educate you on something new.

If you have enjoyed this book and would like to share your positive thoughts, could you please take 30 seconds of your time to go back and give me a review on my Amazon book page.

I greatly appreciate seeing these reviews because it helps me share my hard work.

You can leave me a review on Amazon.com.

Again, thank you and I wish you all the best!

Enjoying this book?

Check out my other best sellers!

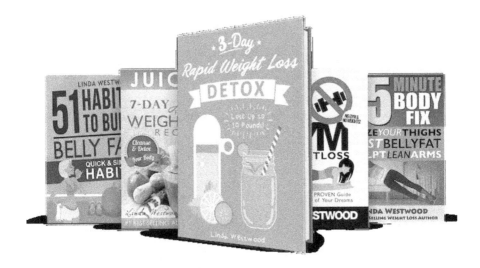

Get your next book on sale here:

TopFitnessAdvice.com/go/books

CPSIA information can be obtained
at www.ICGtesting.com
Printed in the USA
BVHW030615270120
R10616700001B/R106167PG570434BVX1B/1